The Castor Oil Wellness Guide Copy

BERNADETTE LANCE

Contents

CHAPTER ONE

Introduction

What is castor oil?

In the world of natural remedies and holistic wellness, castor oil stands out as a versatile elixir with a rich history and a wide array of applications. This viscous, pale yellow liquid, made from the seeds of the Ricinus communis plant, has been used for ages throughout many civilizations and continents. Castor oil has been ingrained in conventional health, business, and personal care practices since the dawn of civilization and continues to be used in skincare products today.

With its first documented applications in ancient Egypt, where it was a highly valued treatment for constipation and was used in cosmetics and fragrances, castor oil has a long and illustrious history. The ancient Greeks and Romans recognized its medicinal properties, particularly as a purgative, and its influence spread across the Mediterranean. In India, within the framework of Ayurveda, castor oil became integral to traditional healing practices, addressing both internal and external health concerns. The Industrial Revolution marked a transformative period for castor oil, as its non-drying and lubricating qualities found applications in the manufacturing of paints, varnishes, and lubricants. In the modern era, castor oil has experienced a resurgence, aligning with the growing interest in natural remedies and sustainability. Its ancient roots and diverse applications underscore the enduring appeal of castor oil, as it continues to play a multifaceted role in personal care, industry, and holistic health practices.

Adding to the history of castor oil, its application as a multipurpose elixir has crossed national and cultural barriers. Records from ancient China indicate that castor oil was used as a traditional medicine to treat a variety of illnesses, demonstrating the oil's worldwide use. The Middle Ages witnessed the dissemination of knowledge and trade routes that allowed the exchange of goods and ideas, contributing to the continued spread of castor oil's applications.

During the colonial period, castor oil gained prominence in the Americas. Indigenous communities and European settlers alike recognized its medicinal potential, incorporating it into their herbal remedies.

Native American tribes are reported to have used castor oil for its laxative properties and as a salve for skin conditions. Castor oil entered the pharmaceutical sector in the 20th century and was included as a component in a number of different prescription formulations. Its versatility made it a vital component of cosmetic and beauty goods, even outside of the medical field. It is found in products ranging from lip balms to soaps, demonstrating its popularity in skincare routines due to its deep moisturizing and nourishing properties.

Today, the multifaceted nature of castor oil continues to unfold. As an eco-friendly alternative in industries seeking sustainable resources, castor oil has garnered attention for its potential use in bio-based products. Researchers are exploring its applications in biodegradable plastics, further highlighting its role in the ongoing quest for environmentally friendly solutions. The significance of castor oil as a botanical marvel is shown by its ongoing history, which is entrenched in ancient traditions and continuously evolving with modern ideas. Whether used in modern beauty regimens, industrial processes, or traditional medicine, castor oil is proof of the continued value of natural therapies in our constantly changing environment.

CHAPTER TWO

Castor Oil, Your Best Beauty Ally

The capacity of castor oil to offer intense hydration and nourishment is a major factor in its rise to popularity as a beauty product. Packed with fatty acids, particularly the well-known ricinoleic acid, castor oil deeply moisturizes skin and hair follicles. Because of this, it works especially well to fight dryness, flakiness, and dullness, giving the skin and hair a refreshed, glowing appearance. The benefits of castor oil for skincare are numerous. Because of its anti-inflammatory and antibacterial qualities, it's a great option for treating common skin issues. The natural benefits of castor oil include reducing acne and calming irritated skin, which all contribute to a brighter, healthier complexion. Its emollient qualities also aid in diminishing the visibility of wrinkles and fine lines, giving the appearance of more youth. Castor oil has established itself as a go-to remedy for people looking for bright, healthy hair. Hair follicles can be stimulated by regular application on the scalp, which can encourage hair growth. Its nourishing qualities make hair strands stronger and less prone to breakage and broken ends. Particularly well-liked for its ability to treat conditions like alopecia and thinning hair, castor oil provides a healthy substitute for those seeking lush hair.

The benefits of castor oil go beyond improving the appearance of your eyelashes and eyebrows. The moisturizing benefits of the oil on eyelashes may produce a healthier and more voluminous appearance, and its nourishing qualities can help brows grow fuller and thicker. For people who want to accentuate their eye characteristics, castor oil is an affordable and easily applied solution because it can be applied simply with a clean brush.

Castor oil's adaptability is shown in how simple it is to include into different cosmetic routines. Castor oil easily fits into a variety of routines, whether it is applied as a stand-alone therapy, combined with other organic ingredients, or mixed into already-existing skincare and hair care products. It offers a personalized approach to beauty treatment as it may be rubbed into the scalp, blended into DIY masks, or used directly to the face.

CHAPTER THREE

Your Loyal Companion in Your Facial Skin Care

Finding a skincare regimen that is easy to incorporate and effective becomes crucial in the fast-paced world of modern living. Castor oil becomes your faithful friend, making the quest for healthy, glowing facial skin easier to achieve. Making use of castor oil's natural benefits in your daily beauty routine is not only simple but also quite fulfilling. A beauty expert's dream, castor oil offers a simplicity that works well with any skincare regimen. Because of its adaptability, you can use it alone or in combination with other oils to suit your skin's specific requirements. Castor oil easily fits into any lifestyle, whether you're a skincare aficionado with a complex routine or someone looking for simplicity.

Simple yet Effective

Castor oil is a single, elegant act for individuals who appreciate simplicity. Apply a small amount of oil to your damp, clean face and massage it in gently, letting the oil seep into your skin. Rich in fatty acids and other nutrients, its formulation deeply penetrates the skin to leave it feeling renewed and supple. This regimen is a great option for both hectic mornings and leisurely evenings because of its simplicity. The compatibility of castor oil with other oils is what really makes it beautiful. Custom mixes that address the unique requirements of your skin can help you personalize your skincare regimen. For extra hydration, blend it with jojoba oil, or add a drop of lavender oil for a calming, fragrant sensation. The options are as varied as the particular needs of your skin. Castor oil brings out the inner glow when used alone or in well-balanced mixtures. Frequent use helps to promote an even skin tone, minimize blemishes, and minimize fine wrinkles. As it turns into a dependable and constant part of your skincare routine, its loyalty is evident.

Using castor oil goes beyond its amazing skin benefits and becomes a self-care practice. With a moment of calm brought on by the soft massage movements, you may connect with your skin and recognize how easy it is to take care of it. Castor oil's devotion makes taking care of yourself every day an act of self-love. Castor oil shows up in the world of facial skincare products not only as a substance but also as a devoted friend that may effectively and gracefully meet your needs. It is a versatile ally in your journey to vibrant, beautiful skin because it is simple to use into your beauty routine, either on its own or in combination with other oils.

CHAPTER FOUR

Choosing a High-Quality Castor Oil Product

In the crowded field of skincare products, choosing a high-quality castor oil becomes a vital option in assuring best outcomes for your facial skin. An acute attention to detail is necessary to distinguish between the plethora of options available, from extraction techniques to packaging. This is a thorough guide to assist you in choosing the best castor oil product for your beauty routine.

Extraction Methods

Not all castor oils are made equal, and the quality and effectiveness of the oil are greatly influenced by the extraction process. Select goods that use hexane-free or cold-pressed extraction techniques. More of the natural nutrients in cold-pressed castor oil are retained, guaranteeing a higher-quality oil devoid of dangerous compounds. This process maintains the integrity of the oil, providing your skin with a nourishing product full of antioxidants and fatty acids.

Light Protection and the Importance of a Dark Bottle as a Container

Exposure of castor oil to light can have a significant impact on its quality. Select a product that is packaged in a bottle that is dark, amber, or cobalt blue. The oil is shielded from UV radiation that could weaken its efficacy by the dark glass. This guarantees that the potency and effectiveness of the castor oil you use on your face will not diminish from the day it was bottled.

Glass Bottles for Preservation

Picking a dark bottle is important, but so is the container's substance. When choosing castor oil, go for glass bottles rather than plastic ones. Glass keeps potentially dangerous compounds from plastic from leaking into the oil, preserving the product's purity. Because glass is transparent, you can check the oil for color or consistency changes to make sure you're using the best possible product.

Application Precision: The Dropper's Power

A premium castor oil product recognizes the value of application accuracy. Seek out bottles that have a dropper attached. This helps you manage the amount applied, preventing waste and guaranteeing that you use just the proper amount for your skincare routine. It also makes dispensing the oil a breeze. Utilizing a dropper reduces the possibility of contamination, ensuring the potency and purity of your castor oil.

Confidence Certification

Look for castor oil products that are certified organic to add an additional degree of assurance. The oil's organic certification guarantees that it is devoid of pesticides and other dangerous materials, providing a product that is in line with your dedication to clean beauty. Finding premium castor oil requires a discriminating approach. Every little thing, from carefully considered packaging options to extraction techniques that maintain purity, adds to the product's total effectiveness. When you select castor oil that follows these guidelines, you start a skincare journey enhanced by the best natural serum for your face.

CHAPTER FIVE

Facial Skin Care Recipes

There's an amazing universe waiting to be discovered in the center of your kitchen when you set out to improve your skincare regimen. In this chapter, the craft of creating your own skincare elixirs is revealed, with castor oil taking center stage. Take a deep dive into the natural alchemy as we delve into delicious dishes that use castor oil along with other healthy components. These homemade skincare recipes promise to be a soul-satisfying ritual that helps you reconnect with the fundamentals of self-care, in addition to being a delight for your skin. Get ready to experience the enchantment of skincare products blended at home, where each drop reveals a story of radiant beauty and nature turns into your reliable partner in the quest for skin that is bright and revitalized.

CHAPTER SIX

Recipes for Normal Skin

Radiant Glow Facial Elixir with Castor Oil

Ingredients:

1. **Castor oil (1 tablespoon):** This superfood will hydrate and nourish your skin to the core.

2. **Jojoba Oil (1 tablespoon):** Jojoba oil balances oil production and hydrates the skin. It is rich in vitamins E and B.

3. **Rosehip Seed Oil (1 tablespoon):** Rich in antioxidants and

essential fatty acids, rosehip seed oil promotes skin regeneration and fights signs of aging.

4. **Lavender Essential Oil (5 drops):** Known for its calming properties, lavender oil adds a soothing aroma and helps reduce inflammation.

5. **Frankincense Essential Oil (3 drops):** This oil supports skin rejuvenation and may help diminish the appearance of fine lines and wrinkles.

Instructions:

1. **Prepare Your Workspace:** Ensure your workspace is clean, and wash your hands thoroughly before beginning.

2. **Combine Oils:** In a dark glass bottle, combine the castor oil, jojoba oil, and rosehip seed oil. The dark bottle will protect the oils from light, preserving their potency.

3. **Add Essential Oils:** Gently add the drops of lavender and frankincense essential oils to the mixture. These oils not only enhance the scent but also contribute to the overall skincare benefits.

4. **Mix Thoroughly:** Secure the lid on the bottle and shake it well to ensure all the oils are thoroughly mixed. This will create a balanced blend that combines the unique properties of each ingredient.

5. **Patch Test:** Before applying the elixir to your face, perform

a patch test on a small area of skin to ensure you don't have any adverse reactions to the essential oils.

6. **Application:** Use the dropper to dispense a small amount of the elixir onto your fingertips. Gently massage the oil onto your clean, damp face in circular motions, focusing on areas that need extra attention.

7. **Relax and Absorb:** Allow the elixir to absorb into your skin for a few minutes. Take this time to enjoy the calming scents and let the nourishing oils work their magic.

8. **Optional: Warm Compress:** For an extra indulgence, you can place a warm, damp cloth over your face after applying the elixir. This helps open up your pores, allowing the oils to penetrate deeper.

Hydrating Honey & Castor Oil Mask

Ingredients:

1. **Castor Oil (1 tablespoon):** The hydrating foundation of this mask is castor oil, which is well known for its moisturizing qualities.

2. **Raw Honey (1 tablespoon):** Honey, which is rich in antibacterial and antioxidant qualities, helps calm and revitalize skin.

3. **Aloe Vera Gel (1 tablespoon):** Aloe vera gel, well-known for its restorative and cooling qualities, gives the mask a revitalizing touch.

4. **Sweet Almond Oil (1 teaspoon):** Sweet almond oil, which is high in vitamin E, softens and nourishes skin to support a healthy complexion.

5. **Turmeric Powder (1/2 teaspoon):** This anti-inflammatory spice adds a natural glow to the skin and helps even out the complexion.

Instructions:

1. **Mixing the Ingredients:** Aloe vera gel, castor oil, raw honey, sweet almond oil, and turmeric powder should all be combined in a small basin. A smooth, well-blended consis-

tency can be achieved by thoroughly stirring the ingredients.

2. **Patch Test:** Perform a patch test on a small area of skin to ensure there are no allergic reactions to the ingredients, especially if you haven't used turmeric on your skin before.

3. **Application:** Apply the mask evenly to your clean, dry face, avoiding the delicate eye area. Use a gentle, circular motion to massage the mask into your skin.

4. **Relax and Rejuvenate:** Give the mask 15 to 20 minutes to sit on your face. Enjoy this moment to relax and let the healthy components do their job.

5. **Rinse Off:** Gently rinse off the mask with lukewarm water. You may use a soft cloth or your hands to remove the mask thoroughly.

6. **Follow with Moisturizer:** Use your usual moisturizer after patting your skin dry to seal in the moisture and enhance the effects of the mask.

7. **Frequency:** Incorporate this hydrating mask into your skincare routine 1-2 times a week for a refreshing boost of moisture and a radiant complexion.

Balancing Green Tea and Castor Oil Facial Serum for Normal Skin

Ingredients:

1. **Green Tea Infused Oil (2 tablespoons):** Green tea is packed with antioxidants and anti-inflammatory properties, making it ideal for maintaining the balance of normal skin.

2. **Castor Oil (1 tablespoon):** A hydrating and nourishing oil that complements the benefits of green tea for a well-rounded facial serum.

3. **Evening Primrose Oil (1/2 tablespoon):** Known for its gamma-linolenic acid content, evening primrose oil helps maintain skin elasticity and balance.

4. **Geranium Essential Oil (5 drops):** Geranium oil promotes skin balance, helping to regulate oil production and maintain the skin's natural pH.

5. **Vitamin E Oil (1/2 teaspoon):** This antioxidant-rich oil supports skin health and helps protect against environmental damage.

Instructions:

1. **Prepare Green Tea Infused Oil:** Infuse green tea leaves in a carrier oil of your choice (like jojoba or sweet almond oil)

for several hours or overnight. Strain the leaves, leaving you with green tea-infused oil.

2. **Combine Base Oils:** In a dark glass bottle, mix the green tea-infused oil, castor oil, and evening primrose oil. These oils will form the base of your facial serum.

3. **Add Essential Oil:** Integrate the geranium essential oil into the mixture. This oil not only contributes to the serum's balancing properties but also provides a pleasant floral scent.

4. **Include Antioxidant Boost:** Incorporate the vitamin E oil into the serum. Vitamin E acts as a powerful antioxidant, offering additional support to your skin.

5. **Shake Well:** Secure the lid on the bottle and shake it well to ensure all the oils are thoroughly blended, creating a harmonious serum.

6. **Patch Test:** Before applying the serum to your face, perform a patch test on a small area to ensure there are no adverse reactions.

7. **Application:** Dispense a few drops of the serum onto your fingertips and gently massage it onto your clean face, allowing the serum to absorb fully.

8. **Use Daily:** Incorporate this balancing facial serum into your daily skincare routine to maintain the health and harmony of your normal skin.

Rejuvenating Rosehip and Castor Oil Facial Mask for Normal Skin

Ingredients:

1. **Castor Oil (1 tablespoon):** Castor oil, our incredibly nourishing and hydrating oil, serves as the foundation for this restorative mask.

2. **Rosehip Seed Oil (1 tablespoon):** Rosehip seed oil, which is high in vitamins A and C, encourages skin regeneration and enhances the general tone and texture of the skin.

3. **Kaolin Clay (2 tablespoons):** A mild, mineral-rich clay that aids in skin detoxification and cleansing without drying it out too much.

4. **Honey (1 tablespoon):** A natural humectant, honey helps retain moisture, leaving your skin soft and supple.

5. **Lavender Essential Oil (5 drops):** Known for its soothing properties, lavender essential oil adds a calming element to the mask.

Instructions:

1. **Combine Oils and Clay:** Combine the kaolin clay, rosehip seed oil, and castor oil in a bowl. Blend until a smooth, lump-free consistency is reached.

2. **Add Honey:** Incorporate the honey into the mixture. Stir well to ensure even distribution throughout the mask.

3. **Integrate Essential Oil:** Add the drops of lavender essential oil to the mixture. Stir again to disperse the oil evenly.

4. **Patch Test:** Before applying the mask to your face, perform a patch test on a small area to check for any adverse reactions.

5. **Application:** Apply the mask evenly to your clean, dry face, avoiding the eye area. Relax and let the rejuvenating properties of the mask do their work for about 15-20 minutes.

6. **Rinse Off:** Gently rinse the mask off with lukewarm water, using circular motions to exfoliate as you go. Pat your face dry with a clean towel.

7. **Moisturize:** Follow up with your favorite moisturizer to seal in the hydration and leave your skin feeling refreshed.

8. **Frequency:** Use this rejuvenating mask once a week to invigorate and revitalize your normal skin.

Balancing Turmeric and Castor Oil Face Scrub for Normal Skin

Ingredients:

1. **Castor Oil (1 tablespoon):** Renowned for its moisturizing and cleansing properties, castor oil serves as the base of this gentle scrub.

2. **Turmeric Powder (1 teaspoon):** A natural anti-inflammatory and antioxidant, turmeric helps brighten the skin and promote an even tone.

3. **Oatmeal (2 tablespoons, finely ground):** Oatmeal gently exfoliates, soothes, and nourishes the skin, making it perfect for a scrub.

4. **Raw Honey (1 tablespoon):** With its antibacterial properties, honey helps to clarify and hydrate the skin.

5. **Rose Water (1 tablespoon):** Rose water adds a touch of floral freshness while balancing the skin's pH.

Instructions:

1. **Prepare Oatmeal:** Grind the oatmeal into a fine powder using a blender or food processor.

2. **Combine Ingredients:** In a bowl, mix the castor oil,

turmeric powder, finely ground oatmeal, raw honey, and rose water. Stir until you achieve a thick, paste-like consistency.

3. **Patch Test:** Before applying the scrub to your face, perform a patch test on a small area to ensure there are no adverse reactions.

4. **Application:** Gently massage the scrub onto your clean, damp face using circular motions. Focus on areas that may need extra attention, such as the nose and forehead.

5. **Leave on for a Few Minutes:** Allow the scrub to sit on your skin for a few minutes, letting the nourishing properties of the ingredients work their magic.

6. **Rinse Off:** Rinse your face with lukewarm water, using gentle circular motions to exfoliate as you go. Pat your face dry with a clean towel.

7. **Moisturize:** Follow up with your regular moisturizer to keep your skin hydrated after the exfoliation.

8. **Frequency:** Use this balancing turmeric and castor oil face scrub 1-2 times a week to maintain smooth and radiant skin.

Nourishing Avocado and Castor Oil Overnight Mask for Normal Skin

Ingredients:

1. **Avocado (1/2, ripe):** Avocado is rich in vitamins and essential fatty acids, providing deep hydration and nourishment to the skin.

2. **Castor Oil (1 tablespoon):** The moisturizing and replenishing properties of castor oil make it an excellent addition to this overnight mask.

3. **Honey (1 tablespoon):** With its natural humectant properties, honey helps retain moisture, leaving your skin soft and supple.

4. **Yogurt (1 tablespoon, plain):** Yogurt contains lactic acid, which gently exfoliates and brightens the skin.

5. **Lavender Essential Oil (3 drops):** Lavender oil adds a calming aroma while contributing to the overall soothing effects of the mask.

Instructions:

1. **Mash Avocado:** In a bowl, mash half a ripe avocado until it forms a smooth, creamy consistency.

2. **Add Other Ingredients:** Add the castor oil, honey, plain yogurt, and drops of lavender essential oil to the mashed avocado. Mix well until all ingredients are thoroughly combined.

3. **Patch Test:** Before applying the overnight mask to your face, perform a patch test on a small area to ensure there are no adverse reactions.

4. **Application:** Apply the mask evenly to your clean, dry face, avoiding the eye area. Gently massage the mask into your skin using upward motions.

5. **Leave Overnight:** Allow the mask to work its magic overnight. The combination of nourishing ingredients will deeply hydrate and revitalize your skin.

6. **Morning Rinse:** In the morning, rinse your face with lukewarm water to remove the mask. Pat your skin dry with a clean towel.

7. **Moisturize:** Follow up with your regular moisturizer to lock in the hydration and keep your skin feeling nourished throughout the day.

8. **Frequency:** For an extra dose of hydration and regeneration, apply this nutritious nighttime mask made with avocado and castor oil once or twice a week.

This nighttime mask gives normal skin an opulent and intensely nourishing experience by utilizing the power of avocado, castor oil, and other natural ingredients. Your complexion is glowing when you wake up, feeling hydrated, renewed, and prepared to face the day.

Energizing Coffee and Castor Oil Face Scrub for Normal Skin

Ingredients:

1. **Castor Oil (1 tablespoon):** The base of this scrub, castor oil, provides hydration while promoting gentle exfoliation.

2. **Ground Coffee (Half a tablespoon):** Coffee grounds exfoliate the skin, promoting circulation and helping to reveal a brighter complexion.

3. **Coconut Sugar (1 tablespoon):** A natural exfoliant, coconut sugar helps remove dead skin cells, leaving your skin feeling soft and smooth.

4. **Jojoba Oil (1/2 tablespoon):** Jojoba oil helps balance oil production and provides additional hydration without clogging pores.

5. **Vanilla Extract (1/2 teaspoon):** Vanilla not only adds a delightful scent but also contains antioxidants that can soothe and calm the skin.

Instructions:

1. **Combine Dry Ingredients:** In a bowl, mix the ground coffee and coconut sugar. These will serve as the exfoliating agents in your scrub.

2. **Add Wet Ingredients:** Add the castor oil, jojoba oil, and vanilla extract to the dry ingredients. Mix well until all the ingredients are thoroughly combined.

3. **Patch Test:** Before applying the scrub to your face, perform a patch test on a small area to ensure there are no adverse reactions.

4. **Application:** Using circular motions, gently massage the scrub onto your fresh, cleansed face. Concentrate on regions like the nose and forehead that might require more exfoliation.

5. **Leave on for a Few Minutes:** Let the nourishing qualities of the ingredients do their magic on your skin by letting the scrub sit on it for a few minutes.

6. **Rinse Off:** Rinse your face with lukewarm water, using gentle circular motions to exfoliate as you go. Pat your face dry with a clean towel.

7. **Moisturize:** Follow up with your regular moisturizer to keep your skin hydrated after the exfoliation.

8. **Frequency:** Use this energizing coffee and castor oil face scrub 1-2 times a week to maintain smooth and revitalized skin.

Hydrating Olive Oil and Castor Oil Facial Cleansing Oil for Normal Skin

Ingredients:

1. **Castor Oil (1 tablespoon):** Castor oil, the main cleansing agent, aids in the removal of excess oil and pollutants from the skin.

2. **Olive Oil (1 tablespoon):** Olive oil, abundant in antioxidants and moisturizing qualities, lends a refined element to the washing oil.

3. **Grapeseed Oil (1 tablespoon):** Grapeseed oil is lightweight and helps balance oil production, making it suitable for normal skin.

4. **Tea Tree Essential Oil (5 drops):** Known for its antimicrobial properties, tea tree oil helps combat blemishes and keeps the skin clear.

5. **Lemon Essential Oil (3 drops):** Lemon oil brightens the skin and adds a refreshing scent to the cleansing oil.

Instructions:

1. **Prepare Oatmeal:** Grind the oatmeal into a fine powder using a blender or food processor if it's not already finely ground.

2. **Combine Ingredients:** In a bowl, mix the castor oil, finely ground oatmeal, plain yogurt, honey, and drops of lavender essential oil. Stir until you achieve a smooth and consistent mask.

3. **Patch Test:** Before applying the mask to your face, perform a patch test on a small area to ensure there are no adverse reactions.

4. **Application:** Apply the mask evenly to your clean, dry face, avoiding the eye area. Gently massage the mask into your skin using circular motions.

5. **Leave on for 15-20 Minutes:** Allow the mask to sit on your skin for about 15-20 minutes. During this time, the soothing and nourishing properties of the ingredients will work their magic.

6. **Rinse Off:** Gently rinse the mask off with lukewarm water. Use circular motions to exfoliate as you go. Pat your face dry with a clean towel.

7. **Moisturize:** Follow up with your regular moisturizer to lock in the hydration and keep your skin feeling soft and nourished.

8. **Frequency:** Use this soothing oatmeal and castor oil face mask once a week to provide a gentle and calming experience for your normal skin.

Egg Yolk and Castor Oil Hydrating Face Mask for Normal Skin

Ingredients:

1. **Castor Oil (1 tablespoon):** The hydrating and nourishing base, castor oil helps maintain skin health.

2. **Egg Yolk (1):** Egg yolk is rich in vitamins and proteins, promoting skin elasticity and providing a natural lift.

3. **Honey (1 teaspoon):** A natural humectant, honey attracts and retains moisture, leaving the skin hydrated and supple.

4. **Avocado (1 tablespoon, mashed):** Avocado is loaded with healthy fats and antioxidants, contributing to skin nourishment and radiance.

5. **Lemon Juice (1 teaspoon):** Lemon juice helps brighten the skin and balance oil production.

Instructions:

1. **Combine Ingredients:** In a bowl, mix the castor oil, egg yolk, honey, mashed avocado, and lemon juice. Stir until you achieve a smooth and creamy consistency.

2. **Patch Test:** Before applying the mask to your face, perform a patch test on a small area to ensure there are no adverse

reactions.

3. **Application:** Apply the mask evenly to your clean, dry face, avoiding the eye area. Gently massage the mask into your skin using circular motions.

4. **Leave on for 15-20 Minutes:** Allow the mask to sit on your skin for about 15-20 minutes. During this time, the nourishing and hydrating properties of the ingredients will work their magic.

5. **Rinse Off:** Gently rinse the mask off with lukewarm water. Use circular motions to exfoliate as you go. Pat your face dry with a clean towel.

6. **Moisturize:** Follow up with your regular moisturizer to lock in the hydration and keep your skin feeling soft and nourished.

7. **Frequency:** Use this hydrating egg yolk and castor oil face mask once a week to provide a nourishing and revitalizing experience for your normal skin.

CHAPTER SEVEN

Recipes for Sensitive Skin

Soothing Lavender and Chamomile Castor Oil Facial Mist

Ingredients:

1. Distilled Water (1/2 cup): The base of the mist, distilled water provides a clean and pure foundation.

2. Castor Oil (1 tablespoon): A hydrating and nourishing ingredient that forms the core of this facial mist.

3. Lavender Hydrosol (2 tablespoons): Known for its calming

properties, lavender hydrosol adds a soothing and aromatic touch to the mist.

4. Chamomile Essential Oil (5 drops): Chamomile oil is renowned for its anti-inflammatory and skin-soothing properties, making it a perfect addition to this facial mist.

5. Vegetable Glycerin (1/2 teaspoon): Vegetable glycerin helps lock in moisture, keeping your skin hydrated throughout the day.

Instructions:

1. Prepare the Base: In a clean spray bottle, combine the distilled water and castor oil. Shake well to ensure the oil disperses evenly in the water.

2. Add Aromatic Elements: Incorporate the lavender hydrosol and chamomile essential oil into the water and castor oil mixture. These ingredients not only contribute to the mist's soothing properties but also impart a delightful fragrance.

3. Include Moisture-Locking Agent: Add the vegetable glycerin to the mixture. This ingredient helps retain moisture, ensuring that your skin stays hydrated after each misting.

4. Shake Thoroughly: Secure the spray bottle's lid and shake the mixture thoroughly to blend all the ingredients into a harmonious facial mist.

5. Patch Test: Before using the mist on your face, perform a

patch test on a small area to ensure there are no adverse reactions, particularly if you have sensitive skin.

6. Application: Close your eyes and mist your face evenly, holding the spray about 6-8 inches away. Allow the mist to settle on your skin and air dry.

7. Refresh Throughout the Day: Carry the mist with you and refresh your face as needed throughout the day for an instant burst of hydration and tranquility.

Soothing Chamomile and Castor Oil Calming Mask for Normal Skin

Ingredients:

1. **Castor Oil (1 tablespoon):** The key ingredient in this mask, castor oil provides deep hydration and promotes skin health.

2. **Chamomile Tea (1 bag or 1 tablespoon loose):** Chamomile is known for its calming and anti-inflammatory properties, making it perfect for soothing normal skin.

3. **Aloe Vera Gel (1 tablespoon):** Aloe vera is hydrating and helps to reduce inflammation, providing a cooling effect.

4. **Honey (1 teaspoon):** Honey is a natural humectant, attracting and retaining moisture to keep the skin soft and supple.

5. **Lavender Essential Oil (3 drops):** Lavender oil adds a delightful fragrance and contributes to the calming effects of the mask.

Instructions:

1. **Prepare Chamomile Infusion:** Steep the chamomile tea bag or loose chamomile in hot water. Allow it to cool, and then remove the tea bag or strain the loose chamomile, leaving you with chamomile-infused water.

2. **Combine Ingredients:** In a bowl, mix the castor oil, chamomile-infused water, aloe vera gel, honey, and drops of lavender essential oil. Stir well until the ingredients form a smooth and consistent mask.

3. **Patch Test:** Before applying the mask to your face, perform a patch test on a small area to ensure there are no adverse reactions.

4. **Application:** Apply the mask evenly to your clean, dry face, avoiding the eye area. Relax and let the soothing properties of the mask work for about 15-20 minutes.

5. **Rinse Off:** Gently rinse the mask off with lukewarm water. Use circular motions to exfoliate as you go. Pat your face dry with a clean towel.

6. **Moisturize:** Follow up with your regular moisturizer to lock in the hydration and keep your skin feeling calm and nourished.

7. **Frequency:** Use this soothing chamomile and castor oil calming mask once a week or as needed to provide a gentle and calming experience for your normal skin.

Gentle Aloe Vera and Castor Oil Calming Serum for Sensitive Skin

Ingredients:

1. **Castor Oil (1 tablespoon):** The soothing and moisturizing base, castor oil helps nourish sensitive skin without causing irritation.

2. **Aloe Vera Gel (2 tablespoons):** Aloe vera is well-known for its anti-inflammatory and calming properties, making it ideal for sensitive skin.

3. **Chamomile Essential Oil (4 drops):** Chamomile oil adds an extra layer of soothing benefits, reducing redness and calming sensitive skin.

4. **Jojoba Oil (1/2 tablespoon):** Jojoba oil mimics the skin's natural oils, providing gentle hydration without clogging pores.

5. **Vitamin E Oil (1/2 teaspoon):** Vitamin E is an antioxidant that helps protect sensitive skin from environmental stressors.

Instructions:

1. **Combine Base Oils:** In a dark glass bottle, mix the castor oil,

aloe vera gel, jojoba oil, and vitamin E oil. These ingredients create a gentle and nourishing base for the serum.

2. **Add Chamomile Essential Oil:** Incorporate the chamomile essential oil into the mixture. Chamomile's calming properties make it a perfect addition to soothe sensitive skin.

3. **Shake Well:** Secure the lid on the bottle and shake it well to ensure all the oils and aloe vera gel are thoroughly blended, creating a calming serum.

4. **Patch Test:** Before applying the serum to your face, perform a patch test on a small area to ensure there are no adverse reactions.

5. **Application:** Dispense a small amount of the serum onto your fingertips and gently massage it onto your clean face. Allow the serum to absorb fully.

6. **Follow with Moisturizer:** If needed, follow up with a lightweight, fragrance-free moisturizer to lock in the hydration.

7. **Frequency:** Use this gentle aloe vera and castor oil calming serum daily as part of your morning or evening skincare routine to soothe and hydrate sensitive skin.

Soothing Lavender and Calendula Castor Oil Balm for Sensitive Skin

Ingredients:

1. **Castor Oil (2 tablespoons):** The gentle and moisturizing base, castor oil provides a soothing foundation for sensitive skin.

2. **Calendula Infused Oil (1 tablespoon):** Calendula is known for its anti-inflammatory and skin-calming properties, making it excellent for sensitive skin.

3. **Shea Butter (1 tablespoon):** Shea butter is rich in fatty acids and vitamins, providing intense hydration and nourishment.

4. **Lavender Essential Oil (5 drops):** Lavender oil adds a calming and soothing aroma, while also contributing to the balm's skin-soothing properties.

5. **Beeswax (1 tablespoon, grated):** Beeswax helps solidify the balm and provides a protective barrier on the skin.

Instructions:

1. **Prepare Calendula Infused Oil:** Infuse dried calendula flowers in a carrier oil (such as jojoba or sweet almond oil) for several hours or overnight. Strain the flowers, leaving you

with calendula-infused oil.

2. **Melt Ingredients:** In a heat-resistant bowl, combine the castor oil, calendula-infused oil, shea butter, and grated beeswax. Gently melt the ingredients using a double boiler or in short bursts in the microwave.

3. **Add Lavender Essential Oil:** Once melted, remove from heat and let it cool slightly. Add the drops of lavender essential oil and stir well to incorporate the calming fragrance.

4. **Pour into Container:** Pour the mixture into a clean, airtight container. Allow it to cool and solidify.

5. **Patch Test:** Before applying the balm to your face, perform a patch test on a small area to ensure there are no adverse reactions.

6. **Application:** Scoop a small amount of the balm with clean fingers and gently apply it to sensitive areas on your face. Focus on areas that may need extra care or experience redness.

7. **Use as Needed:** Apply the soothing balm as needed throughout the day, especially when your skin requires extra comfort and hydration.

8. **Storage:** Store the balm in a cool, dark place to maintain its consistency and effectiveness.

This calming balm combines the soothing properties of castor oil, calendula, and lavender to provide relief for sensitive skin. Shea butter and beeswax contribute to a rich and protective formulation, creating a gentle balm that helps maintain the delicate balance of sensitive skin.

Gentle Almond and Castor Oil Cleansing Milk for Sensitive Skin

Ingredients:

1. **Castor Oil (1 tablespoon):** The soothing and cleansing base, castor oil helps remove impurities without irritating sensitive skin.

2. **Sweet Almond Oil (2 tablespoons):** Almond oil is gentle, lightweight, and rich in vitamins, providing nourishment without clogging pores.

3. **Aloe Vera Gel (1 tablespoon):** Aloe vera is renowned for its anti-inflammatory properties, offering a cooling and calming effect for sensitive skin.

4. **Rose Water (2 tablespoons):** Rose water is gentle and helps balance the skin's pH while providing a subtle floral scent.

5. **Lavender Essential Oil (3 drops):** Lavender oil adds a calming aroma and contributes to the overall soothing effects of the cleansing milk.

Instructions:

1. **Combine Base Oils:** In a dark glass bottle, mix the castor oil and sweet almond oil. These oils create a nourishing and cleansing blend suitable for sensitive skin.

2. **Add Aloe Vera and Rose Water:** Integrate the aloe vera

gel and rose water into the oil mixture. These ingredients provide additional soothing and hydrating benefits.

3. **Include Lavender Essential Oil:** Add the drops of lavender essential oil to the mixture. Stir well to disperse the oil evenly and enhance the cleansing milk's calming properties.

4. **Shake Well:** Secure the lid on the bottle and shake it well before each use to ensure all the ingredients are thoroughly blended.

5. **Patch Test:** Before using the cleansing milk on your face, perform a patch test on a small area to ensure there are no adverse reactions.

6. **Application:** Dispense a small amount of the cleansing milk onto a cotton pad or your fingertips and gently massage it onto your dry face. Use circular motions to lift away impurities.

7. **Rinse Off or Remove:** You can either rinse your face with lukewarm water or use a damp cotton pad to gently wipe away the cleansing milk. Pat your face dry with a clean towel.

8. **Follow with Moisturizer:** If needed, follow up with a fragrance-free, hypoallergenic moisturizer to keep your skin hydrated.

9. **Frequency:** Use this gentle almond and castor oil cleansing milk as part of your daily skincare routine, both morning and evening, to cleanse and soothe sensitive skin.

This cleansing milk combines the gentle cleansing properties of castor and almond oil with the soothing effects of aloe vera, rose water, and lavender essential oil. It provides a mild and effective way to cleanse sensitive skin without causing irritation, leaving your skin feeling clean, calm, and cared for.

Soothing Jojoba and Castor Oil Facial Serum for Sensitive Skin

Ingredients:

1. **Castor Oil (1 tablespoon):** The calming and moisturizing base, castor oil helps soothe sensitive skin without causing irritation.

2. **Jojoba Oil (2 tablespoons):** Jojoba oil closely resembles the skin's natural sebum, providing gentle hydration and nourishment.

3. **Calendula Infused Oil (1 tablespoon):** Calendula is known for its anti-inflammatory properties, making it ideal for calming sensitive skin.

4. **Chamomile Essential Oil (4 drops):** Chamomile oil adds extra soothing benefits and reduces redness in sensitive skin.

5. **Rosehip Seed Oil (1/2 teaspoon):** Rich in vitamins A and C, rosehip seed oil helps promote skin regeneration and improve overall skin health.

Instructions:

1. **Prepare Calendula Infused Oil:** Infuse dried calendula flowers in a carrier oil (such as jojoba or sweet almond oil) for several hours or overnight. Strain the flowers, leaving you

with calendula-infused oil.

2. **Combine Base Oils:** In a dark glass bottle, mix the castor oil, jojoba oil, and calendula-infused oil. These oils create a nourishing and calming serum for sensitive skin.

3. **Add Chamomile Essential Oil:** Incorporate the chamomile essential oil into the mixture. Chamomile's soothing properties make it an excellent addition for sensitive skin.

4. **Include Rosehip Seed Oil:** Add the rosehip seed oil to the serum. This oil enhances the serum's skin-regenerating properties.

5. **Shake Well:** Secure the lid on the bottle and shake it well before each use to ensure all the ingredients are thoroughly blended.

6. **Patch Test:** Before applying the serum to your face, perform a patch test on a small area to ensure there are no adverse reactions.

7. **Application:** Dispense a small amount of the serum onto your fingertips and gently press it onto your clean face. Allow the serum to absorb fully.

8. **Follow with Moisturizer:** If needed, follow up with a hypoallergenic moisturizer to lock in the hydration and keep your sensitive skin comfortable.

9. **Frequency:** Use this soothing jojoba and castor oil facial serum twice daily as part of your skincare routine to nourish

and calm sensitive skin.

This serum combines the gentle and calming properties of castor and jojoba oil with the soothing effects of calendula and chamomile. The addition of rosehip seed oil promotes skin regeneration, making it a comprehensive solution for sensitive skin in need of extra care and hydration.

Soothing Marshmallow Extract and Castor Oil Facial Cream for Sensitive Skin

Ingredients:

1. **Castor Oil (1.5 tablespoons):** The soothing and moisturizing base, castor oil helps calm sensitive skin and provides deep hydration.

2. **Marshmallow Extract (1 tablespoon):** Marshmallow extract is known for its anti-inflammatory and skin-soothing properties, making it ideal for sensitive skin.

3. **Sweet Almond Oil (1 tablespoon):** Almond oil is gentle, lightweight, and rich in vitamins, providing nourishment without clogging pores.

4. **Shea Butter (1 tablespoon):** Shea butter is deeply moisturizing and helps create a protective barrier on sensitive skin.

5. **Calendula Essential Oil (5 drops):** Calendula oil adds extra soothing benefits and promotes skin comfort for sensitive skin.

Instructions:

1. **Combine Base Ingredients:** In a heat-resistant bowl, mix the castor oil, marshmallow extract, sweet almond oil, and shea butter.

2. **Create a Double Boiler:** Set up a double boiler by placing the bowl over a pot of simmering water. Gently heat the ingredients until the shea butter melts, stirring to combine.

3. **Cool Slightly:** Allow the mixture to cool slightly before adding the calendula essential oil. Stir well to incorporate the soothing aroma.

4. **Transfer to Container:** Once the cream has reached a comfortable temperature, transfer it to a clean, airtight container. Let it cool and solidify.

5. **Patch Test:** Before applying the cream to your face, perform a patch test on a small area to ensure there are no adverse reactions.

6. **Application:** Scoop a small amount of the cream with clean fingertips and gently apply it to your sensitive skin. Massage in circular motions until fully absorbed.

7. **Use as Needed:** Apply the soothing cream as needed throughout the day, especially when your skin requires extra comfort and hydration.

8. **Storage:** Store the cream in a cool, dark place to maintain its consistency and effectiveness.

Soothing Cucumber and Castor Oil Cooling Mask for Sensitive Skin

Ingredients:

1. **Castor Oil (1 tablespoon):** The calming and moisturizing base, castor oil helps soothe sensitive skin without causing irritation.

2. **Cucumber (1/2, peeled and grated):** Cucumber is known for its cooling and anti-inflammatory properties, making it ideal for sensitive skin.

3. **Oat Flour (2 tablespoons):** Oat flour is gentle and helps soothe sensitive skin while providing a soft, creamy texture to the mask.

4. **Greek Yogurt (1 tablespoon):** Greek yogurt is rich in pro-biotics and lactic acid, offering a calming and hydrating effect.

5. **Chamomile Essential Oil (3 drops):** Chamomile oil adds extra soothing benefits and promotes relaxation.

Instructions:

1. **Grate Cucumber:** Peel and grate half a cucumber to extract its soothing properties.

2. **Combine Ingredients:** In a bowl, mix the castor oil, grated cucumber, oat flour, Greek yogurt, and drops of chamomile essential oil. Stir until you achieve a smooth and consistent mask.

3. **Patch Test:** Before applying the mask to your face, perform a patch test on a small area to ensure there are no adverse reactions.

4. **Application:** Apply the mask evenly to your clean, dry face, avoiding the eye area. Relax and let the cooling and soothing properties of the mask work for about 15-20 minutes.

5. **Rinse Off:** Gently rinse the mask off with lukewarm water. Use circular motions to exfoliate as you go. Pat your face dry with a clean towel.

6. **Moisturize:** Follow up with a hypoallergenic, fragrance-free moisturizer to lock in the hydration and keep your sensitive skin feeling calm and nourished.

7. **Frequency:** Use this soothing cucumber and castor oil cooling mask once a week or as needed to provide a gentle and calming experience for your sensitive skin.

Soothing Rosewater and Castor Oil Face Mist for Sensitive Skin

Ingredients:

1. **Castor Oil (1 tablespoon):** The calming and moisturizing base, castor oil helps soothe sensitive skin without causing irritation.

2. **Rosewater (1/4 cup):** Rosewater is gentle and known for its anti-inflammatory properties, making it perfect for calming and hydrating sensitive skin.

3. **Aloe Vera Gel (1 tablespoon):** Aloe vera provides additional soothing and hydrating benefits, helping to maintain the skin's moisture balance.

4. **Vegetable Glycerin (1 teaspoon):** Vegetable glycerin is a humectant that attracts moisture to the skin, promoting hydration without clogging pores.

5. **Lavender Essential Oil (4 drops):** Lavender oil adds a calming aroma and contributes to the overall soothing effects of the mist.

Instructions:

1. **Combine Ingredients:** In a small spray bottle, mix the castor oil, rosewater, aloe vera gel, vegetable glycerin, and drops

of lavender essential oil. Shake well to ensure all the ingredients are thoroughly blended.

2. **Patch Test:** Before using the face mist on your entire face, perform a patch test on a small area to ensure there are no adverse reactions.

3. **Application:** Close your eyes and lightly mist your face with the soothing mixture. Hold the bottle about 8-10 inches away from your face for an even application.

4. **Allow to Dry:** Allow the mist to air dry or gently pat it into your skin with clean fingertips.

5. **Use Throughout the Day:** Spritz the mist on your face whenever your sensitive skin needs a refreshing and calming boost. It's suitable for use throughout the day.

6. **Storage:** Store the face mist in a cool, dark place and shake well before each use to ensure the ingredients remain well-mixed.

The calming effects of castor oil, rosewater, aloe vera, and lavender essential oil are combined in this peaceful face spray. It offers sensitive skin a mild and moisturizing solution that promotes a sensation of relaxation and refreshment whenever needed.

Tea Tree and Castor Oil Clarifying Facial Cleanser for Sensitive Skin

Ingredients:

1. **Castor Oil (1.5 tablespoons):** The calming and moisturizing base, castor oil helps soothe sensitive skin without causing irritation.

2. **Jojoba Oil (1 tablespoon):** Jojoba oil closely resembles the skin's natural oils, providing gentle hydration without clogging pores.

3. **Tea Tree Essential Oil (7 drops):** Tea tree oil is known for its antibacterial and clarifying properties, making it suitable for sensitive skin prone to blemishes.

4. **Chamomile Infusion (1/4 cup):** Chamomile is soothing and anti-inflammatory, providing a calming effect for sensitive skin.

5. **Aloe Vera Gel (1 tablespoon):** Aloe vera provides additional soothing and hydrating benefits, helping to maintain the skin's moisture balance.

Instructions:

1. **Prepare Chamomile Infusion:** Steep chamomile tea in hot water and allow it to cool. Strain the tea, leaving you with

chamomile-infused water.

2. **Combine Base Ingredients:** In a dark glass bottle, mix the castor oil, jojoba oil, chamomile infusion, and aloe vera gel. Shake well to ensure all ingredients are thoroughly blended.

3. **Add Tea Tree Essential Oil:** Incorporate the drops of tea tree essential oil into the mixture. Shake the bottle again to evenly distribute the tea tree oil.

4. **Patch Test:** Before using the cleanser on your face, perform a patch test on a small area to ensure there are no adverse reactions.

5. **Application:** Dispense a small amount of the cleanser onto a cotton pad or your fingertips. Gently massage it onto your damp face in circular motions.

6. **Rinse Off:** Rinse your face with lukewarm water, ensuring all the cleanser is removed. Pat your face dry with a clean towel.

7. **Moisturize:** Follow up with a fragrance-free, hypoallergenic moisturizer to keep your sensitive skin hydrated.

8. **Frequency:** Use this clarifying tea tree and castor oil facial cleanser daily as part of your skincare routine, both morning and evening, to keep your sensitive skin clear and balanced.

CHAPTER EIGHT

Recipes for Dry Skin

Gentle Mango and Castor Oil Nourishing Balm for Dry Skin

Ingredients:

1. **Castor Oil (1.5 tablespoons):** The calming and moisturizing base, castor oil helps soothe sensitive skin without causing irritation.

2. **Mango Butter (1 tablespoon):** Mango butter is rich in fatty acids and vitamins, providing deep nourishment and a protective barrier for sensitive skin.

3. **Calendula Infused Oil (1 tablespoon):** Calendula is known for its anti-inflammatory properties, making it ideal

for calming and soothing sensitive skin.

4. **Jojoba Oil (1/2 tablespoon):** Jojoba oil closely resembles the skin's natural oils, providing gentle hydration without clogging pores.

5. **Lavender Essential Oil (4 drops):** Lavender oil adds a calming aroma and contributes to the overall soothing effects of the balm.

Instructions:

1. **Prepare Calendula Infused Oil:** Infuse dried calendula flowers in a carrier oil (such as jojoba or sweet almond oil) for several hours or overnight. Strain the flowers, leaving you with calendula-infused oil.

2. **Combine Base Ingredients:** In a heat-resistant bowl, mix the castor oil, mango butter, calendula-infused oil, and jojoba oil.

3. **Create a Double Boiler:** Set up a double boiler by placing the bowl over a pot of simmering water. Gently heat the ingredients until the mango butter melts, stirring to combine.

4. **Cool Slightly:** Allow the mixture to cool slightly before adding the drops of lavender essential oil. Stir well to incorporate the calming fragrance.

5. **Transfer to Container:** Once the balm has reached a comfortable temperature, transfer it to a clean, airtight container. Allow it to cool and solidify.

6. **Patch Test:** Before applying the balm to your face, perform a patch test on a small area to ensure there are no adverse reactions.

7. **Application:** Scoop a small amount of the balm with clean fingers and gently apply it to sensitive areas on your face. Massage in circular motions until fully absorbed.

8. **Use as Needed:** Apply the nourishing balm as needed throughout the day, especially when your skin requires extra comfort and hydration.

9. **Storage:** Store the balm in a cool, dark place to maintain its consistency and effectiveness.

This nourishing balm combines the calming properties of castor oil, mango butter, and calendula, providing a rich and protective solution for sensitive skin. The addition of jojoba oil and lavender essential oil enhances the balm's soothing effects, leaving your skin feeling moisturized, calm, and cared for.

Nourishing Castor and Argan Oil Hydrating Face Serum for Dry Skin

Ingredients:

1. **Castor Oil (1.5 tablespoons):** The deeply moisturizing base, castor oil helps replenish dry skin and provides essential hydration.

2. **Argan Oil (1.5 tablespoons):** Argan oil is rich in antioxidants and fatty acids, promoting nourishment and preventing dryness.

3. **Rosehip Seed Oil (1/2 teaspoon):** Rosehip seed oil aids in skin regeneration, helping to improve the texture of dry skin.

4. **Vitamin E Oil (1/2 teaspoon):** Vitamin E is an antioxidant that supports skin health and helps combat dryness.

5. **Lavender Essential Oil (4 drops):** Lavender oil adds a soothing aroma and contributes to the overall hydrating effects of the serum.

Instructions:

1. **Combine Base Oils:** In a dark glass bottle, mix the castor oil, argan oil, rosehip seed oil, and vitamin E oil. These oils create a rich and nourishing base for the serum.

2. **Add Lavender Essential Oil:** Incorporate the drops of lavender essential oil into the mixture. Gently shake the bottle to ensure the oils are thoroughly blended.

3. **Patch Test:** Before applying the serum to your face, perform a patch test on a small area to ensure there are no adverse reactions.

4. **Application:** Dispense a small amount of the serum onto your fingertips and gently press it onto your clean, dry face. Allow the serum to absorb fully.

5. **Follow with Moisturizer:** If needed, follow up with a rich, hydrating moisturizer to lock in the nourishment and keep your dry skin feeling supple.

6. **Frequency:** Use this nourishing castor and argan oil hydrating serum daily as part of your evening skincare routine to deeply hydrate and revitalize dry skin.

This serum combines the deeply moisturizing properties of castor and argan oil with the skin-regenerating effects of rosehip seed oil and vitamin E. The addition of lavender essential oil adds a touch of relaxation, creating a luxurious and hydrating experience for dry skin.

Moisturizing Castor and Wheat Germ Oil Face Mask for Dry Skin

Ingredients:

1. **Castor Oil (1 tablespoon):** The deeply moisturizing base, castor oil helps replenish dry skin and provides essential hydration.

2. **Wheat Germ Oil (1 tablespoon):** Wheat germ oil is rich in vitamins A and E, promoting nourishment and preventing dryness.

3. **Honey (1 tablespoon):** Honey is a natural humectant, attracting and retaining moisture to keep dry skin hydrated.

4. **Banana (1/2, ripe):** Banana is packed with vitamins and minerals, providing additional nourishment and promoting a soft, smooth complexion.

5. **Yogurt (1 tablespoon):** Yogurt contains lactic acid, offering gentle exfoliation and contributing to skin renewal.

Instructions:

1. **Mash the Banana:** In a bowl, mash half a ripe banana until it forms a smooth consistency.

2. **Add Castor and Wheat Germ Oil:** Add the castor oil and

wheat germ oil to the mashed banana. Stir well to combine the ingredients.

3. **Incorporate Honey:** Pour in the honey and mix thoroughly. Honey adds extra moisturizing benefits and helps create a spreadable mask.

4. **Include Yogurt:** Add the yogurt to the mixture. Yogurt contributes to the mask's creamy texture and provides gentle exfoliation.

5. **Mix Well:** Stir all the ingredients together until you achieve a uniform and smooth mask.

6. **Patch Test:** Before applying the mask to your face, perform a patch test on a small area to ensure there are no adverse reactions.

7. **Application:** Apply the mask evenly to your clean, dry face, avoiding the eye area. Relax and let the mask sit for about 15-20 minutes.

8. **Rinse Off:** Gently rinse the mask off with lukewarm water. Use circular motions to exfoliate as you go. Pat your face dry with a clean towel.

9. **Moisturize:** Follow up with a rich, hydrating moisturizer to lock in the nourishment and keep your dry skin feeling soft and supple.

10. **Frequency:** Use this moisturizing castor and wheat germ oil face mask once a week to deeply hydrate and revitalize dry skin, promoting a radiant complexion.

Avocado and Castor Oil Deep Hydration Facial Balm for Dry Skin

Ingredients:

1. **Castor Oil (1.5 tablespoons):** The deeply moisturizing base, castor oil helps replenish dry skin and provides essential hydration.

2. **Avocado Oil (1.5 tablespoons):** Avocado oil is rich in fatty acids and vitamins, offering deep nourishment to dry skin.

3. **Shea Butter (1 tablespoon):** Shea butter is deeply moisturizing and helps create a protective barrier on dry skin.

4. **Beeswax (1 tablespoon, grated):** Beeswax helps solidify the balm and provides a protective layer to lock in moisture.

5. **Vitamin E Oil (1/2 teaspoon):** Vitamin E is an antioxidant that supports skin health and helps combat dryness.

Instructions:

1. **Melt Ingredients:** In a heat-resistant bowl, combine the castor oil, avocado oil, shea butter, grated beeswax, and vitamin E oil. Gently melt the ingredients using a double boiler or in short bursts in the microwave.

2. **Stir Well:** Stir the mixture well to ensure all the ingredients are thoroughly combined. Allow it to cool slightly.

3. **Pour into Container:** Once the balm has reached a comfortable temperature, pour it into a clean, airtight container. Let it cool and solidify.

4. **Patch Test:** Before applying the balm to your face, perform a patch test on a small area to ensure there are no adverse reactions.

5. **Application:** Scoop a small amount of the balm with clean fingers and gently apply it to your dry skin. Massage in circular motions until fully absorbed.

6. **Use as Needed:** Apply the deep hydration balm as needed throughout the day, especially when your skin requires extra comfort and hydration.

7. **Storage:** Store the balm in a cool, dark place to maintain its consistency and effectiveness.

Soothing Coconut and Castor Oil Moisturizing Cream for Dry Skin

Ingredients:

1. **Castor Oil (1.5 tablespoons):** The deeply moisturizing base, castor oil helps replenish dry skin and provides essential hydration.

2. **Coconut Oil (1.5 tablespoons):** Coconut oil is rich in fatty acids, offering deep nourishment and a pleasant tropical aroma.

3. **Cocoa Butter (1 tablespoon):** Cocoa butter is highly moisturizing and helps create a protective barrier on dry skin.

4. **Almond Oil (1 tablespoon):** Almond oil is lightweight and rich in vitamins, providing additional nourishment without clogging pores.

5. **Vanilla Extract (1/2 teaspoon):** Vanilla extract adds a delightful fragrance to the cream.

Instructions:

1. **Melt Ingredients:** In a heat-resistant bowl, combine the castor oil, coconut oil, cocoa butter, almond oil, and vanilla extract. Gently melt the ingredients using a double boiler or in short bursts in the microwave.

2. **Stir Well:** Stir the mixture well to ensure all the ingredients are thoroughly combined. Allow it to cool slightly.

3. **Transfer to Container:** Once the cream has reached a comfortable temperature, transfer it to a clean, airtight container. Let it cool and solidify.

4. **Patch Test:** Before applying the cream to your face, perform a patch test on a small area to ensure there are no adverse reactions.

5. **Application:** Scoop a small amount of the cream with clean fingers and gently apply it to your dry skin. Massage in circular motions until fully absorbed.

6. **Use as Needed:** Apply the moisturizing cream as needed throughout the day, especially when your skin requires extra comfort and hydration.

7. **Storage:** Store the cream in a cool, dark place to maintain its consistency and effectiveness.

Hydrating Shea Butter and Castor Oil Face Mask for Dry Skin

Ingredients:

1. **Castor Oil (1.5 tablespoons):** The deeply moisturizing base, castor oil helps replenish dry skin and provides essential hydration.

2. **Shea Butter (1.5 tablespoons):** Shea butter is highly moisturizing and helps create a protective barrier on dry skin.

3. **Honey (1 tablespoon):** Honey is a natural humectant, attracting and retaining moisture to keep dry skin hydrated.

4. **Avocado (1/4, mashed):** Avocado is rich in fatty acids and vitamins, offering deep nourishment and promoting skin elasticity.

5. **Lavender Essential Oil (4 drops):** Lavender oil adds a calming aroma and contributes to the overall soothing effects of the mask.

Instructions:

1. **Combine Base Oils:** In a dark glass bottle, mix the castor oil, vitamin E oil, sweet almond oil, and rosehip seed oil. These oils create a potent and nourishing blend.

2. **Add Lavender Essential Oil:** Incorporate the drops of lavender essential oil into the mixture. Gently shake the bottle to ensure the oils are thoroughly blended.

3. **Patch Test:** Before applying the serum to your face, perform a patch test on a small area to ensure there are no adverse reactions.

4. **Application:** Before bedtime, dispense a small amount of the serum onto your fingertips and gently massage it onto your clean, dry face. Allow the serum to absorb fully.

5. **Follow with Night Cream:** If needed, follow up with a rich night cream to lock in the nourishment and keep your dry skin feeling supple.

6. **Frequency:** Use this revitalizing vitamin E and castor oil night serum as part of your nightly skincare routine to deeply hydrate and rejuvenate dry skin.

Rejuvenating Camellia and Castor Oil Facial Moisturizer for Dry Skin

Ingredients:

1. **Castor Oil (1.5 tablespoons):** The deeply moisturizing base, castor oil helps replenish dry skin and provides essential hydration.

2. **Camellia Oil (1.5 tablespoons):** Camellia oil is rich in antioxidants and fatty acids, offering deep nourishment and promoting skin elasticity.

3. **Shea Butter (1 tablespoon):** Shea butter is highly moisturizing and helps create a protective barrier on dry skin.

4. **Argan Oil (1/2 teaspoon):** Argan oil is rich in vitamins and antioxidants, providing additional nourishment without clogging pores.

5. **Geranium Essential Oil (3 drops):** Geranium oil is known for its skin-balancing properties and adds a floral aroma to the moisturizer.

Instructions:

1. **Combine Base Ingredients:** In a heat-resistant bowl, mix the castor oil, camellia oil, shea butter, and argan oil. Gently heat the ingredients until the shea butter melts, stirring to

combine.

2. **Cool Slightly:** Allow the mixture to cool slightly before adding the drops of geranium essential oil. Stir well to incorporate the floral fragrance.

3. **Transfer to Container:** Once the moisturizer has reached a comfortable temperature, transfer it to a clean, airtight container. Allow it to cool and solidify.

4. **Patch Test:** Before applying the moisturizer to your face, perform a patch test on a small area to ensure there are no adverse reactions.

5. **Application:** Scoop a small amount of the moisturizer with clean fingers and gently apply it to your dry skin. Massage in circular motions until fully absorbed.

6. **Use as Needed:** Apply the rejuvenating moisturizer as needed throughout the day, especially when your skin requires extra comfort and hydration.

7. **Storage:** Store the moisturizer in a cool, dark place to maintain its consistency and effectiveness.

Restorative Bakuchiol and Castor Oil Facial Serum for Dry Skin

Ingredients:

1. **Castor Oil (1 tablespoon):** The deeply moisturizing base, castor oil helps replenish dry skin and provides essential hydration.

2. **Bakuchiol Oil (1 tablespoon):** Bakuchiol is a natural alternative to retinol, known for its anti-aging and skin-restoring properties.

3. **Jojoba Oil (1/2 tablespoon):** Jojoba oil closely resembles the skin's natural oils, providing gentle hydration without clogging pores.

4. **Rosehip Seed Oil (1/2 teaspoon):** Rosehip seed oil aids in skin regeneration, helping to improve the texture of dry skin.

5. **Frankincense Essential Oil (3 drops):** Frankincense oil is known for its skin-regenerating properties and adds a subtle, calming aroma.

Instructions:

1. **Combine Base Oils:** In a dark glass bottle, mix the castor oil, bakuchiol oil, jojoba oil, and rosehip seed oil. These oils create a powerful and rejuvenating serum.

2. **Add Frankincense Essential Oil:** Incorporate the drops of frankincense essential oil into the mixture. Gently shake the

bottle to ensure the oils are thoroughly blended.

3. **Patch Test:** Before applying the serum to your face, perform a patch test on a small area to ensure there are no adverse reactions.

4. **Application:** Dispense a small amount of the serum onto your fingertips and gently press it onto your clean, dry face. Allow the serum to absorb fully.

5. **Follow with Moisturizer:** If needed, follow up with a rich, hydrating moisturizer to lock in the nourishment and keep your dry skin feeling supple.

6. **Frequency:** Use this restorative bakuchiol and castor oil facial serum as part of your evening skincare routine to target dryness and promote a revitalized complexion.

Hydrating Apricot Kernel and Castor Oil Facial Elixir for Dry Skin

Ingredients:

1. **Castor Oil (1.5 tablespoons):** The deeply moisturizing base, castor oil helps replenish dry skin and provides essential hydration.

2. **Apricot Kernel Oil (1.5 tablespoons):** Apricot kernel oil is rich in fatty acids and vitamins, offering deep nourishment and promoting skin suppleness.

3. **Shea Butter (1 tablespoon):** Shea butter is highly moisturizing and helps create a protective barrier on dry skin.

4. **Calendula Infused Oil (1/2 teaspoon):** Calendula is known for its anti-inflammatory properties, making it ideal for calming and soothing dry skin.

5. **Lavender Essential Oil (4 drops):** Lavender oil adds a calming aroma and contributes to the overall soothing effects of the elixir.

Instructions:

1. **Combine Base Oils:** In a dark glass bottle, mix the castor oil, apricot kernel oil, shea butter, and calendula infused oil. These oils create a rich and nourishing elixir.

2. **Add Lavender Essential Oil:** Incorporate the drops of lavender essential oil into the mixture. Gently shake the bottle to ensure the oils are thoroughly blended.

3. **Patch Test:** Before applying the elixir to your face, perform a patch test on a small area to ensure there are no adverse reactions.

4. **Application:** Dispense a small amount of the elixir onto your fingertips and gently press it onto your clean, dry face. Allow the elixir to absorb fully.

5. **Follow with Moisturizer:** If needed, follow up with a rich, hydrating moisturizer to lock in the nourishment and keep your dry skin feeling supple.

6. **Frequency:** Use this hydrating apricot kernel and castor oil facial elixir daily as part of your skincare routine to deeply moisturize and revitalize dry skin.

CHAPTER NINE

Recipes for Oily Skin

Balancing Squalane and Castor Oil Facial Serum for Oily Skin

Ingredients:

1. **Castor Oil (1 tablespoon):** Though castor oil is often associated with dry skin, it can help balance oil production and cleanse pores.

2. **Squalane Oil (1.5 tablespoons):** Squalane is a lightweight oil that hydrates without clogging pores, making it suitable for oily skin.

3. **Jojoba Oil (1/2 tablespoon):** Jojoba oil closely resembles the skin's natural oils, providing gentle hydration without promoting excess oiliness.

4. **Tea Tree Essential Oil (5 drops):** Tea tree oil is known for

its antibacterial properties, making it beneficial for oily skin prone to breakouts.

5. **Lemon Essential Oil (3 drops):** Lemon oil has astringent properties that can help control excess oil on the skin.

Instructions:

1. **Combine Base Oils:** In a dark glass bottle, mix the castor oil, squalane oil, and jojoba oil. These oils create a lightweight and balancing serum for oily skin.

2. **Add Essential Oils:** Incorporate the drops of tea tree essential oil and lemon essential oil into the mixture. Gently shake the bottle to ensure the oils are thoroughly blended.

3. **Patch Test:** Before applying the serum to your face, perform a patch test on a small area to ensure there are no adverse reactions.

4. **Application:** Dispense a small amount of the serum onto your fingertips and gently press it onto your clean, damp face. Allow the serum to absorb fully.

5. **Follow with Moisturizer (if needed):** Depending on your skin's needs, you can follow up with a lightweight, oil-free moisturizer.

6. **Frequency:** Use this balancing squalane and castor oil facial serum daily as part of your skincare routine to help regulate oil production and maintain a balanced complexion.

Mattifying Sunflower Seed and Castor Oil Facial Serum for Oily Skin

Ingredients:

1. **Castor Oil (1 tablespoon):** Castor oil helps balance oil production and cleanse pores, making it beneficial for oily skin.

2. **Sunflower Seed Oil (1.5 tablespoons):** Sunflower seed oil is lightweight and rich in linoleic acid, known for its non-comedogenic properties, making it suitable for oily skin.

3. **Grapeseed Oil (1/2 tablespoon):** Grapeseed oil is a light and easily absorbed oil that helps control oil production without clogging pores.

4. **Lavender Essential Oil (4 drops):** Lavender oil adds a calming aroma and contributes to the overall soothing effects of the serum.

5. **Tea Tree Essential Oil (3 drops):** Tea tree oil is known for its antibacterial properties, making it beneficial for oily skin prone to breakouts.

Instructions:

1. **Combine Base Oils:** In a dark glass bottle, mix the castor

oil, sunflower seed oil, and grapeseed oil. These oils create a lightweight and mattifying serum for oily skin.

2. **Add Essential Oils:** Incorporate the drops of lavender essential oil and tea tree essential oil into the mixture. Gently shake the bottle to ensure the oils are thoroughly blended.

3. **Patch Test:** Before applying the serum to your face, perform a patch test on a small area to ensure there are no adverse reactions.

4. **Application:** Dispense a small amount of the serum onto your fingertips and gently press it onto your clean, damp face. Allow the serum to absorb fully.

5. **Follow with Moisturizer (if needed):** Depending on your skin's needs, you can follow up with a lightweight, oil-free moisturizer.

6. **Frequency:** Use this mattifying sunflower seed and castor oil facial serum daily as part of your skincare routine to help regulate oil production and maintain a matte complexion.

This serum combines the benefits of castor oil and sunflower seed oil to control oil production and maintain a matte finish on oily skin. Grapeseed oil further contributes to the serum's lightweight texture, while lavender and tea tree essential oils provide soothing and antibacterial properties. Regular use can help balance oily skin, reduce breakouts, and leave your skin feeling refreshed.

Balancing Grapeseed and Castor Oil Facial Tonic for Oily Skin

Ingredients:

1. **Castor Oil (1 tablespoon):** Castor oil helps regulate oil production and cleanse pores, making it beneficial for oily skin.

2. **Grapeseed Oil (1.5 tablespoons):** Grapeseed oil is lightweight and rich in linoleic acid, known for its non-comedogenic properties, making it suitable for oily skin.

3. **Rosemary Essential Oil (4 drops):** Rosemary oil is known for its astringent properties, helping to tone and balance oily skin.

4. **Lemon Essential Oil (3 drops):** Lemon oil has astringent properties that can help control excess oil on the skin.

5. **Geranium Essential Oil (2 drops):** Geranium oil helps balance sebum production and adds a pleasant floral aroma.

Instructions:

1. **Combine Base Oils:** In a dark glass bottle, mix the castor oil and grapeseed oil. These oils create a lightweight and balancing tonic for oily skin.

2. **Add Essential Oils:** Incorporate the drops of rosemary essential oil, lemon essential oil, and geranium essential oil into the mixture. Gently shake the bottle to ensure the oils are thoroughly blended.

3. **Patch Test:** Before applying the tonic to your face, perform a patch test on a small area to ensure there are no adverse reactions.

4. **Application:** Dispense a small amount of the tonic onto a cotton pad and gently sweep it across your clean, damp face. Allow the tonic to air dry.

5. **Follow with Moisturizer (if needed):** Depending on your skin's needs, you can follow up with a lightweight, oil-free moisturizer.

6. **Frequency:** Use this balancing grapeseed and castor oil facial tonic daily as part of your skincare routine to help regulate oil production and maintain a balanced complexion.

Harmonizing Ylang Ylang and Castor Oil Facial Elixir for Oily Skin

Ingredients:

1. **Castor Oil (1 tablespoon):** Castor oil helps regulate oil production and cleanse pores, making it beneficial for oily skin.

2. **Jojoba Oil (1.5 tablespoons):** Jojoba oil closely resembles the skin's natural oils, providing gentle hydration without clogging pores.

3. **Grapeseed Oil (1/2 tablespoon):** Grapeseed oil is lightweight and rich in linoleic acid, known for its non-comedogenic properties, making it suitable for oily skin.

4. **Ylang Ylang Essential Oil (4 drops):** Ylang ylang oil helps balance sebum production and adds a sweet floral aroma.

Instructions:

1. **Combine Base Oils:** In a dark glass bottle, mix the castor oil, jojoba oil, and grapeseed oil. These oils create a lightweight and balancing elixir for oily skin.

2. **Add Ylang Ylang Essential Oil:** Incorporate the drops of ylang ylang essential oil into the mixture. Gently shake the bottle to ensure the oils are thoroughly blended.

3. **Patch Test:** Before applying the elixir to your face, perform a patch test on a small area to ensure there are no adverse reactions.

4. **Application:** Dispense a small amount of the elixir onto your fingertips and gently press it onto your clean, damp face. Allow the elixir to absorb fully.

5. **Follow with Moisturizer (if needed):** Depending on your skin's needs, you can follow up with a lightweight, oil-free moisturizer.

6. **Frequency:** Use this harmonizing ylang ylang and castor oil facial elixir daily as part of your skincare routine to help regulate oil production and maintain a balanced complexion.

Purifying Myrrh and Castor Oil Facial Serum for Oily Skin

Ingredients:

1. **Castor Oil (1 tablespoon):** Castor oil helps regulate oil production and cleanse pores, making it beneficial for oily skin.

2. **Argan Oil (1.5 tablespoons):** Argan oil is rich in vitamins and antioxidants, providing additional nourishment without clogging pores.

3. **Safflower Seed Oil (1/2 tablespoon):** Safflower seed oil is lightweight and helps balance oil production on the skin.

4. **Myrrh Essential Oil (3 drops):** Myrrh oil is known for its purifying properties and adds a warm, earthy aroma.

Instructions:

1. **Combine Base Oils:** In a dark glass bottle, mix the castor oil, argan oil, and safflower seed oil. These oils create a lightweight and purifying serum for oily skin.

2. **Add Myrrh Essential Oil:** Incorporate the drops of myrrh essential oil into the mixture. Gently shake the bottle to ensure the oils are thoroughly blended.

3. **Patch Test:** Before applying the serum to your face, perform a patch test on a small area to ensure there are no adverse reactions.

4. **Application:** Dispense a small amount of the serum onto your fingertips and gently press it onto your clean, damp face. Allow the serum to absorb fully.

5. **Follow with Moisturizer (if needed):** Depending on your skin's needs, you can follow up with a lightweight, oil-free moisturizer.

6. **Frequency:** Use this purifying myrrh and castor oil facial serum daily as part of your skincare routine to help regulate oil production and promote a clearer complexion.

Balancing Sea Moss and Castor Oil Facial Serum for Oily Skin

Ingredients:

1. **Castor Oil (1 tablespoon):** Castor oil helps regulate oil production and cleanse pores, making it beneficial for oily skin.

2. **Sea Moss Gel (1.5 tablespoons):** Sea moss is rich in minerals and can help balance excess oil on the skin.

3. **Grapeseed Oil (1/2 tablespoon):** Grapeseed oil is lightweight and rich in linoleic acid, known for its non-comedogenic properties, making it suitable for oily skin.

4. **Tea Tree Essential Oil (4 drops):** Tea tree oil is known for its antibacterial properties, making it beneficial for oily skin prone to breakouts.

Instructions:

1. **Prepare Sea Moss Gel:** If you don't have pre-made sea moss gel, you can prepare it by blending soaked sea moss with water until you get a smooth, gel-like consistency.

2. **Combine Base Oils and Sea Moss Gel:** In a dark glass bottle, mix the castor oil, grapeseed oil, and sea moss gel. These ingredients create a lightweight and balancing serum

for oily skin.

3. **Add Tea Tree Essential Oil:** Incorporate the drops of tea tree essential oil into the mixture. Gently shake the bottle to ensure the oils and sea moss gel are thoroughly blended.

4. **Patch Test:** Before applying the serum to your face, perform a patch test on a small area to ensure there are no adverse reactions.

5. **Application:** Dispense a small amount of the serum onto your fingertips and gently press it onto your clean, damp face. Allow the serum to absorb fully.

6. **Follow with Moisturizer (if needed):** Depending on your skin's needs, you can follow up with a lightweight, oil-free moisturizer.

7. **Frequency:** Use this balancing sea moss and castor oil facial serum daily as part of your skincare routine to help regulate oil production and maintain a balanced complexion.

Clarifying Lemon and Castor Oil Facial Tonic for Oily Skin

Ingredients:

1. **Castor Oil (1 tablespoon):** Castor oil helps regulate oil production and cleanse pores, making it beneficial for oily skin.

2. **Lemon Juice (1.5 tablespoons):** Lemon juice contains citric acid, which helps to clarify and balance oily skin.

3. **Jojoba Oil (1/2 tablespoon):** Jojoba oil closely resembles the skin's natural oils, providing gentle hydration without promoting excess oiliness.

4. **Lavender Essential Oil (4 drops):** Lavender oil adds a calming aroma and contributes to the overall soothing effects of the tonic.

Instructions:

1. **Combine Base Ingredients:** In a dark glass bottle, mix the castor oil, lemon juice, and jojoba oil. These ingredients create a clarifying tonic for oily skin.

2. **Add Lavender Essential Oil:** Incorporate the drops of lavender essential oil into the mixture. Gently shake the bottle to ensure the ingredients are thoroughly blended.

3. **Patch Test:** Before applying the tonic to your face, perform a patch test on a small area to ensure there are no adverse reactions.

4. **Application:** Dispense a small amount of the tonic onto a cotton pad and gently sweep it across your clean, damp face. Allow the tonic to air dry.

5. **Follow with Moisturizer (if needed):** Depending on your skin's needs, you can follow up with a lightweight, oil-free moisturizer.

6. **Caution:** Lemon juice may increase sensitivity to sunlight. It's advisable to use this tonic in the evening and apply sunscreen during the day.

7. **Frequency:** Use this clarifying lemon and castor oil facial tonic every other day as part of your skincare routine to help control excess oil and maintain a balanced complexion.

Balancing Sage and Castor Oil Facial Serum for Oily Skin

Ingredients:

1. **Castor Oil (1 tablespoon):** Castor oil helps regulate oil production and cleanse pores, making it beneficial for oily skin.

2. **Grapeseed Oil (1.5 tablespoons):** Grapeseed oil is lightweight and rich in linoleic acid, known for its non-comedogenic properties, making it suitable for oily skin.

3. **Sage Essential Oil (4 drops):** Sage oil has astringent properties and can help balance sebum production on oily skin.

4. **Tea Tree Essential Oil (3 drops):** Tea tree oil is known for its antibacterial properties, making it beneficial for oily skin prone to breakouts.

Instructions:

1. **Combine Base Oils:** In a dark glass bottle, mix the castor oil and grapeseed oil. These oils create a lightweight and balancing serum for oily skin.

2. **Add Essential Oils:** Incorporate the drops of sage essential oil and tea tree essential oil into the mixture. Gently shake the bottle to ensure the oils are thoroughly blended.

3. **Patch Test:** Before applying the serum to your face, perform a patch test on a small area to ensure there are no adverse reactions.

4. **Application:** Dispense a small amount of the serum onto your fingertips and gently press it onto your clean, damp face. Allow the serum to absorb fully.

5. **Follow with Moisturizer (if needed):** Depending on your skin's needs, you can follow up with a lightweight, oil-free moisturizer.

6. **Frequency:** Use this balancing sage and castor oil facial serum daily as part of your skincare routine to help regulate oil production and maintain a balanced complexion.

Purifying Witch Hazel and Castor Oil Facial Tonic for Oily Skin

Ingredients:

1. **Castor Oil (1 tablespoon):** Castor oil helps regulate oil production and cleanse pores, making it beneficial for oily skin.

2. **Witch Hazel (1.5 tablespoons):** Witch hazel is a natural astringent that helps tone and clarify oily skin.

3. **Grapeseed Oil (1/2 tablespoon):** Grapeseed oil is lightweight and rich in linoleic acid, known for its non-comedogenic properties, making it suitable for oily skin.

4. **Lemon Essential Oil (4 drops):** Lemon oil has astringent properties that can help control excess oil on the skin.

Instructions:

1. **Combine Base Ingredients:** In a dark glass bottle, mix the castor oil, witch hazel, and grapeseed oil. These ingredients create a purifying tonic for oily skin.

2. **Add Lemon Essential Oil:** Incorporate the drops of lemon essential oil into the mixture. Gently shake the bottle to ensure the ingredients are thoroughly blended.

3. **Patch Test:** Before applying the tonic to your face, perform a patch test on a small area to ensure there are no adverse reactions.

4. **Application:** Dispense a small amount of the tonic onto a cotton pad and gently sweep it across your clean, damp face. Allow the tonic to air dry.

5. **Follow with Moisturizer (if needed):** Depending on your skin's needs, you can follow up with a lightweight, oil-free moisturizer.

6. **Caution:** Lemon oil may increase sensitivity to sunlight. It's advisable to use this tonic in the evening and apply sunscreen during the day.

7. **Frequency:** Use this purifying witch hazel and castor oil facial tonic every other day as part of your skincare routine to help control excess oil and maintain a balanced complexion.

Detoxifying Charcoal and Castor Oil Facial Mask for Oily Skin

Ingredients:

1. **Activated Charcoal Powder (1 tablespoon):** Activated charcoal helps absorb excess oil, impurities, and toxins from the skin.

2. **Castor Oil (1.5 tablespoons):** Castor oil helps regulate oil production and cleanse pores, making it beneficial for oily skin.

3. **Aloe Vera Gel (1 tablespoon):** Aloe vera has soothing properties and helps hydrate the skin without adding extra oil.

4. **Tea Tree Essential Oil (5 drops):** Tea tree oil is known for its antibacterial properties, making it beneficial for oily skin prone to breakouts.

Instructions:

1. **Prepare the Mask:** In a non-metallic bowl, mix the activated charcoal powder, castor oil, aloe vera gel, and tea tree essential oil. Stir well until you achieve a smooth paste.

2. **Patch Test:** Before applying the mask to your face, perform a patch test on a small area to ensure there are no adverse

reactions.

3. **Application:** Using a clean brush or your fingertips, apply an even layer of the mask to your clean, damp face, avoiding the eye and mouth area.

4. **Relax:** Allow the mask to dry for 15-20 minutes. During this time, the charcoal will work to draw out impurities and excess oil from your skin.

5. **Rinse Off:** Once the mask is dry, gently rinse it off with lukewarm water. Pat your face dry with a clean towel.

6. **Follow with Moisturizer (if needed):** Depending on your skin's needs, you can follow up with a lightweight, oil-free moisturizer.

7. **Frequency:** Use this charcoal and castor oil facial mask once or twice a week as part of your skincare routine to help detoxify and balance oily skin.

CHAPTER TEN

Body Care Recipes

Nourishing Castor Oil Body Scrub for Silky Smooth Skin

Ingredients:

1. **Castor Oil (2 tablespoons):** Castor oil is deeply moisturizing and helps soften and nourish the skin.

2. **Brown Sugar (1/2 cup):** Brown sugar provides gentle exfoliation, removing dead skin cells and promoting smoother skin.

3. **Coconut Oil (2 tablespoons):** Coconut oil adds additional hydration and imparts a delightful tropical scent.

4. **Vanilla Extract (1 teaspoon):** Vanilla extract adds a sweet

aroma and enhances the overall scent of the scrub.

Instructions:

1. **Combine Ingredients:** In a bowl, mix together the castor oil, brown sugar, coconut oil, and vanilla extract until well combined.

2. **Test Consistency:** Adjust the sugar and oil proportions if needed until you achieve a scrub with a thick, spreadable consistency.

3. **Shower Preparation:** Before applying the scrub, ensure your body is wet and ready for exfoliation. Stand in the shower or bath.

4. **Application:** Scoop a small amount of the scrub onto your fingertips and gently massage it onto your skin using circular motions. Focus on areas prone to roughness, like elbows, knees, and heels.

5. **Rinse Off:** Rinse off the scrub thoroughly with warm water, allowing the oils to leave a nourishing layer on your skin.

6. **Pat Dry:** Gently pat your skin dry with a towel. Avoid rubbing too vigorously to allow the oils to remain on your skin.

7. **Optional Moisturization:** If desired, follow up with your favorite body lotion or more castor oil for added moisture.

8. **Frequency:** Use this nourishing castor oil body scrub once or twice a week to maintain smooth and supple skin.

This DIY body scrub combines the moisturizing properties of castor oil with the exfoliating benefits of brown sugar and the hydrating effects of coconut oil. The addition of vanilla extract enhances the sensory experience, leaving your skin silky smooth and delicately scented.

Ultra-Moisturizing Shea Butter and Castor Oil Body Balm

Ingredients:

1. **Shea Butter (1/2 cup):** Shea butter is rich in fatty acids and vitamins, providing deep hydration to the skin.

2. **Castor Oil (1/4 cup):** Castor oil adds a thicker consistency and additional moisturizing benefits to the body balm.

3. **Sweet Almond Oil (1/4 cup):** Sweet almond oil is lightweight and absorbs easily, enhancing the overall moisturizing properties.

4. **Lavender Essential Oil (10-15 drops):** Lavender oil not only adds a calming fragrance but also contributes to the soothing effects on the skin.

Instructions:

1. **Melt Shea Butter and Oils:** In a double boiler or a heat-safe bowl over simmering water, melt the shea butter, castor oil, and sweet almond oil until they form a liquid.

2. **Cool Slightly:** Allow the melted mixture to cool slightly but not solidify completely.

3. **Add Lavender Essential Oil:** Once slightly cooled, stir in

the lavender essential oil for a soothing fragrance. Adjust the number of drops based on your preference.

4. **Blend Well:** Mix the ingredients thoroughly to ensure an even distribution of oils and fragrance.

5. **Transfer to Jar:** Pour the liquid balm into a clean, airtight jar or container.

6. **Cool and Solidify:** Allow the body balm to cool and solidify at room temperature or in the refrigerator.

7. **Application:** Scoop a small amount of the balm and massage it onto your body, paying extra attention to dry areas.

8. **Use After Bath or Shower:** For best results, apply the body balm on damp skin after a bath or shower to lock in moisture.

9. **Frequency:** Use this ultra-moisturizing shea butter and castor oil body balm as needed to keep your skin deeply nourished and hydrated.

Rich Cocoa Butter and Castor Oil Body Lotion

Ingredients:

1. **Cocoa Butter (1/2 cup):** Cocoa butter is deeply moisturizing and helps improve skin elasticity.

2. **Castor Oil (1/4 cup):** Castor oil provides additional nourishment and helps keep the skin hydrated.

3. **Coconut Oil (1/4 cup):** Coconut oil adds a light texture and enhances the overall moisturizing properties.

4. **Vanilla Extract (1 teaspoon):** Vanilla extract adds a sweet aroma and complements the natural chocolate scent of cocoa butter.

Instructions:

1. **Melt Cocoa Butter and Oils:** In a double boiler or a heat-safe bowl over simmering water, melt the cocoa butter, castor oil, and coconut oil until they form a liquid.

2. **Cool Slightly:** Allow the melted mixture to cool slightly but not solidify completely.

3. **Add Vanilla Extract:** Once slightly cooled, stir in the vanilla extract for a sweet fragrance. Mix well.

4. **Blend Thoroughly:** Use a whisk or hand mixer to blend

the ingredients thoroughly, ensuring a smooth and creamy consistency.

5. **Transfer to Container:** Pour the lotion into a clean, airtight container or pump bottle.

6. **Cool and Set:** Allow the body lotion to cool and set at room temperature or in the refrigerator.

7. **Application:** Dispense a small amount of the lotion and apply it to your body, massaging gently until absorbed.

8. **Use After Bath or Shower:** For best results, apply the body lotion on damp skin after a bath or shower to lock in moisture.

9. **Frequency:** Use this rich cocoa butter and castor oil body lotion daily to maintain soft, nourished, and delicately scented skin.

Tip: This body lotion is perfect for stretch marks! It combines the richness of cocoa butter with the moisturizing benefits of castor oil, creating a luxurious and deeply nourishing experience for your skin.

Soothing Illipe Butter and Castor Oil Body Butter

Ingredients:

1. **Illipe Butter (1/2 cup):** Illipe butter is rich in fatty acids and promotes deep moisturization, leaving the skin feeling soft and supple.

2. **Castor Oil (1/4 cup):** Castor oil adds additional nourishment and helps retain moisture in the skin.

3. **Jojoba Oil (1/4 cup):** Jojoba oil closely resembles the skin's natural oils, providing hydration without a greasy feel.

4. **Chamomile Essential Oil (10 drops):** Chamomile oil has soothing properties, making it ideal for calming and comforting the skin.

Instructions:

1. **Melt Illipe Butter and Oils:** In a double boiler or a heat-safe bowl over simmering water, melt the illipe butter, castor oil, and jojoba oil until they form a liquid.

2. **Cool Slightly:** Allow the melted mixture to cool slightly but not solidify completely.

3. **Add Chamomile Essential Oil:** Once slightly cooled, stir in the chamomile essential oil for a soothing fragrance. Mix

well.

4. **Blend Thoroughly:** Use a hand mixer or whisk to blend the ingredients thoroughly, ensuring a smooth and creamy consistency.

5. **Transfer to Jar:** Pour the body butter into a clean, airtight jar or container.

6. **Cool and Set:** Allow the body butter to cool and set at room temperature or in the refrigerator.

7. **Application:** Scoop a small amount of the body butter and massage it onto your body, focusing on areas prone to dryness.

8. **Use After Bath or Shower:** For best results, apply the body butter on damp skin after a bath or shower to lock in moisture.

9. **Frequency:** Use this soothing illipe butter and castor oil body butter as needed to keep your skin deeply nourished and hydrated.

Revitalizing Galbanum and Castor Oil Body Oil

Ingredients:

1. **Castor Oil (1/2 cup):** Castor oil provides deep moisturization and helps improve skin elasticity.

2. **Sweet Almond Oil (1/4 cup):** Sweet almond oil is lightweight and absorbs easily, adding additional hydration to the skin.

3. **Grapeseed Oil (1/4 cup):** Grapeseed oil is rich in antioxidants and promotes skin health while maintaining a non-greasy feel.

4. **Galbanum Essential Oil (10 drops):** Galbanum oil has a fresh, green aroma and is believed to have revitalizing properties for the skin.

Instructions:

1. **Combine Base Oils:** In a dark glass bottle, mix the castor oil, sweet almond oil, and grapeseed oil. These oils create a nourishing base for the body oil.

2. **Add Galbanum Essential Oil:** Incorporate the drops of galbanum essential oil into the mixture. Gently shake the bottle to ensure the oils are thoroughly blended.

3. **Patch Test:** Before applying the body oil to your skin, perform a patch test on a small area to ensure there are no adverse reactions.

4. **Application:** Dispense a small amount of the body oil onto your palms and massage it onto your body, focusing on areas that need extra care.

5. **Use After Bath or Shower:** For best results, apply the body oil on damp skin after a bath or shower to lock in moisture.

6. **Enjoy the Aroma:** Take a moment to enjoy the refreshing and revitalizing aroma of galbanum essential oil as you apply the body oil.

7. **Frequency:** Use this revitalizing galbanum and castor oil body oil as part of your daily body care routine to promote skin hydration and a sense of renewal.

Hydrating Flaxseed Mucilage and Castor Oil Body Gel

Ingredients:

1. **Flaxseed Mucilage (1/2 cup):** Flaxseed mucilage is rich in omega-3 fatty acids and has hydrating properties for the skin.

2. **Castor Oil (1/4 cup):** Castor oil provides deep moisturization and helps maintain skin elasticity.

3. **Argan Oil (1/4 cup):** Argan oil is rich in vitamins and antioxidants, contributing to overall skin health.

4. **Lavender Essential Oil (10 drops):** Lavender oil adds a calming and soothing fragrance to the body gel.

Instructions:

1. **Prepare Flaxseed Mucilage:** To make flaxseed mucilage, boil flaxseeds in water until it forms a gel-like consistency. Strain to obtain the mucilage.

2. **Combine Ingredients:** In a bowl, mix the flaxseed mucilage, castor oil, argan oil, and lavender essential oil until well combined.

3. **Adjust Consistency:** If needed, adjust the ratio of flaxseed mucilage to achieve the desired gel-like consistency.

4. **Transfer to Container:** Pour the body gel into a clean,

airtight container or pump bottle.

5. **Application:** Dispense a small amount of the body gel and massage it onto your body, focusing on areas that need hydration.

6. **Use After Bath or Shower:** For best results, apply the body gel on damp skin after a bath or shower to lock in moisture.

7. **Enjoy the Fragrance:** Allow the calming aroma of lavender essential oil to enhance your sensory experience during application.

8. **Frequency:** Use this hydrating flaxseed mucilage and castor oil body gel daily or as needed to maintain skin hydration and promote a soothing effect.

Nourishing Murumuru Butter and Castor Oil Body Cream

Ingredients:

1. **Murumuru Butter (1/2 cup):** Murumuru butter is rich in fatty acids, promoting deep hydration and improving skin texture.

2. **Castor Oil (1/4 cup):** Castor oil provides additional moisturization and helps retain skin elasticity.

3. **Coconut Oil (1/4 cup):** Coconut oil adds a light texture and enhances the overall nourishing properties of the body cream.

4. **Ylang Ylang Essential Oil (10 drops):** Ylang ylang oil adds a sweet floral fragrance and is believed to have calming effects on the skin.

Instructions:

1. **Melt Murumuru Butter and Oils:** In a double boiler or a heat-safe bowl over simmering water, melt the murumuru butter, castor oil, and coconut oil until they form a liquid.

2. **Cool Slightly:** Allow the melted mixture to cool slightly but not solidify completely.

3. **Add Ylang Ylang Essential Oil:** Once slightly cooled, stir in the ylang ylang essential oil for a floral fragrance. Mix well.

4. **Blend Thoroughly:** Use a hand mixer or whisk to blend the ingredients thoroughly, ensuring a creamy and smooth consistency.

5. **Transfer to Jar:** Pour the body cream into a clean, airtight jar or container.

6. **Cool and Set:** Allow the body cream to cool and set at room temperature or in the refrigerator.

7. **Application:** Scoop a small amount of the body cream and massage it onto your body, paying attention to areas prone to dryness.

8. **Use After Bath or Shower:** For best results, apply the body cream on damp skin after a bath or shower to lock in moisture.

9. **Enjoy the Fragrance:** Allow the sweet floral aroma of ylang ylang to add a touch of indulgence to your body care routine.

10. **Frequency:** Use this nourishing murumuru butter and castor oil body cream daily to keep your skin deeply moisturized, smooth, and delicately scented.

Soothing Tagetes Oil and Castor Oil Body Balm

Ingredients:

1. **Castor Oil (1/2 cup):** Castor oil provides deep moisturization and helps improve skin elasticity.

2. **Shea Butter (1/4 cup):** Shea butter is rich in fatty acids and vitamins, contributing to intense hydration and nourishment.

3. **Jojoba Oil (1/4 cup):** Jojoba oil closely resembles the skin's natural oils, offering additional hydration without a greasy feel.

4. **Tagetes Essential Oil (10 drops):** Tagetes oil has a sweet and citrusy aroma, believed to have soothing and calming effects on the skin.

Instructions:

1. **Melt Shea Butter and Oils:** In a double boiler or a heat-safe bowl over simmering water, melt the shea butter, castor oil, and jojoba oil until they form a liquid.

2. **Cool Slightly:** Allow the melted mixture to cool slightly but not solidify completely.

3. **Add Tagetes Essential Oil:** Once slightly cooled, stir in the

tagetes essential oil for a sweet and citrusy fragrance. Mix well.

4. **Blend Thoroughly:** Use a hand mixer or whisk to blend the ingredients thoroughly, ensuring a smooth and creamy consistency.

5. **Transfer to Jar:** Pour the body balm into a clean, airtight jar or container.

6. **Cool and Set:** Allow the body balm to cool and set at room temperature or in the refrigerator.

7. **Application:** Scoop a small amount of the body balm and massage it onto your body, focusing on areas that need extra care.

8. **Use After Bath or Shower:** For best results, apply the body balm on damp skin after a bath or shower to lock in moisture.

9. **Enjoy the Aroma:** Let the sweet and citrusy scent of tagetes oil enhance your sensory experience during application.

10. **Frequency:** Use this soothing tagetes oil and castor oil body balm as needed to maintain skin hydration and enjoy its calming effects.

Relaxing Lavender Oil and Castor Oil Body Lotion for Sleep

Ingredients:

1. **Castor Oil (1/2 cup):** Castor oil provides deep moisturization, promoting soft and supple skin.

2. **Cocoa Butter (1/4 cup):** Cocoa butter is rich in antioxidants and adds a luxurious feel, nourishing the skin.

3. **Sweet Almond Oil (1/4 cup):** Sweet almond oil is lightweight and easily absorbed, contributing to overall skin hydration.

4. **Lavender Essential Oil (15 drops):** Lavender oil is renowned for its calming and relaxing properties, promoting a peaceful sleep.

Instructions:

1. **Melt Cocoa Butter and Oils:** In a double boiler or a heat-safe bowl over simmering water, melt the cocoa butter, castor oil, and sweet almond oil until they form a liquid.

2. **Cool Slightly:** Allow the melted mixture to cool slightly but not solidify completely.

3. **Add Lavender Essential Oil:** Once slightly cooled, stir in

the lavender essential oil for a soothing and sleep-inducing fragrance. Mix well.

4. **Blend Thoroughly:** Use a hand mixer or whisk to blend the ingredients thoroughly, ensuring a smooth and creamy consistency.

5. **Transfer to Jar:** Pour the body lotion into a clean, airtight jar or container.

6. **Cool and Set:** Allow the body lotion to cool and set at room temperature or in the refrigerator.

7. **Application:** Before bedtime, apply a generous amount of the body lotion onto your body, focusing on areas that benefit from extra hydration.

8. **Relaxing Bedtime Routine:** Incorporate the application of this body lotion into your nightly routine as a calming ritual before sleep.

9. **Enjoy a Peaceful Sleep:** Allow the soothing scent of lavender to help create a tranquil atmosphere, contributing to a restful night's sleep.

10. **Frequency:** Use this relaxing lavender oil and castor oil body lotion as part of your bedtime routine to promote relaxation and improve the overall quality of your sleep.

Revitalizing Orange Oil and Castor Oil Body Scrub for Morning Energization

Ingredients:

1. **Castor Oil (1/2 cup):** Castor oil provides deep moisturization, leaving your skin soft and hydrated.

2. **Coconut Oil (1/4 cup):** Coconut oil adds a light texture and enhances the overall nourishing properties of the body scrub.

3. **Granulated Sugar (1/2 cup):** Granulated sugar provides gentle exfoliation, removing dead skin cells for a smoother complexion.

4. **Orange Essential Oil (15 drops):** Orange oil has a refreshing and invigorating fragrance, revitalizing the senses in the morning.

Instructions:

1. **Melt Coconut Oil:** In a microwave-safe bowl, melt the coconut oil until it becomes a liquid.

2. **Combine Ingredients:** In a mixing bowl, combine the melted coconut oil, castor oil, granulated sugar, and orange essential oil. Mix well until you achieve a consistent scrub.

3. **Test Consistency:** Adjust the sugar and oil proportions if needed until you achieve a scrub with a thick, spreadable consistency.

4. **Transfer to Container:** Pour the body scrub into a clean, airtight jar or container.

5. **Cool and Set:** Allow the body scrub to cool and set at room temperature.

6. **Application:** In the morning, take a small amount of the body scrub and massage it onto damp skin in gentle circular motions. Focus on areas that need revitalization.

7. **Rinse Off:** Rinse off the scrub thoroughly with warm water, leaving your skin feeling refreshed.

8. **Pat Dry:** Gently pat your skin dry with a towel. Avoid rubbing too vigorously to allow the oils to remain on your skin.

9. **Enjoy the Aroma:** Allow the invigorating scent of orange essential oil to awaken your senses and prepare you for the day ahead.

10. **Frequency:** Use this revitalizing orange oil and castor oil body scrub a few times a week in the morning to start your day with refreshed and energized skin.

Soothing Oat Milk and Castor Oil Body Lotion

Ingredients:

1. **Castor Oil (1/2 cup):** Castor oil provides deep moisturization, promoting soft and supple skin.

2. **Oat Milk (1/4 cup):** Oat milk is soothing and nourishing, known for its calming effects on the skin.

3. **Shea Butter (1/4 cup):** Shea butter is rich in fatty acids and vitamins, contributing to intense hydration and nourishment.

4. **Vanilla Extract (1 teaspoon):** Vanilla extract adds a sweet aroma, enhancing the overall sensory experience.

Instructions:

1. **Melt Shea Butter and Oils:** In a double boiler or a heat-safe bowl over simmering water, melt the shea butter and castor oil until they form a liquid.

2. **Cool Slightly:** Allow the melted mixture to cool slightly but not solidify completely.

3. **Add Oat Milk and Vanilla Extract:** Once slightly cooled, stir in the oat milk and vanilla extract. Mix well to incorporate all ingredients.

4. **Blend Thoroughly:** Use a hand mixer or whisk to blend the ingredients thoroughly, ensuring a smooth and creamy consistency.

5. **Transfer to Jar:** Pour the body lotion into a clean, airtight jar or container.

6. **Cool and Set:** Allow the body lotion to cool and set at room temperature or in the refrigerator.

7. **Application:** After a bath or shower, apply a generous amount of the body lotion onto your body, focusing on areas that need extra care.

8. **Enjoy the Aroma:** Let the sweet scent of vanilla and the soothing properties of oat milk envelop your senses.

9. **Frequency:** Use this soothing oat milk and castor oil body lotion daily to keep your skin deeply moisturized, soft, and delicately scented.

Nourishing Evening Primrose and Castor Oil Body Oil

Ingredients:

1. **Castor Oil (1/2 cup):** Castor oil provides deep moisturization, promoting soft and supple skin.

2. **Evening Primrose Oil (1/4 cup):** Evening primrose oil is rich in gamma-linolenic acid, known for its nourishing and skin-soothing properties.

3. **Jojoba Oil (1/4 cup):** Jojoba oil closely resembles the skin's natural oils, offering additional hydration without a greasy feel.

4. **Lavender Essential Oil (10 drops):** Lavender oil adds a calming fragrance and complements the overall soothing effects of evening primrose oil.

Instructions:

1. **Combine Base Oils:** In a dark glass bottle, mix the castor oil, evening primrose oil, and jojoba oil. These oils create a nourishing base for the body oil.

2. **Add Lavender Essential Oil:** Incorporate the drops of lavender essential oil into the mixture. Gently shake the bottle to ensure the oils are thoroughly blended.

3. **Patch Test:** Before applying the body oil to your skin, perform a patch test on a small area to ensure there are no adverse reactions.

4. **Application:** Dispense a small amount of the body oil onto your palms and massage it onto your body, focusing on areas that need extra care.

5. **Use After Bath or Shower:** For best results, apply the body oil on damp skin after a bath or shower to lock in moisture.

6. **Enjoy the Fragrance:** Take a moment to enjoy the calming aroma of lavender essential oil as you apply the body oil.

7. **Frequency:** Use this nourishing evening primrose and castor oil body oil as part of your daily body care routine to promote skin hydration and a sense of tranquility.

This body oil combines the moisturizing benefits of castor oil, evening primrose oil, and jojoba oil with the calming properties of lavender essential oil. Pamper your skin with this aromatic blend to leave it feeling deeply nourished, hydrated, and delicately scented.

Hydrating Pumpkin Seed Oil and Castor Oil Body Butter

Ingredients:

1. **Castor Oil (1/2 cup):** Castor oil provides deep moisturization, leaving your skin soft and hydrated.

2. **Pumpkin Seed Oil (1/4 cup):** Pumpkin seed oil is rich in antioxidants and essential fatty acids, offering nourishing benefits for the skin.

3. **Cocoa Butter (1/4 cup):** Cocoa butter adds a luxurious feel and enhances the overall moisturizing properties of the body butter.

4. **Cinnamon Essential Oil (10 drops):** Cinnamon oil adds a warm and inviting fragrance while promoting a sense of comfort.

Instructions:

1. **Melt Cocoa Butter and Oils:** In a double boiler or a heat-safe bowl over simmering water, melt the cocoa butter and castor oil until they form a liquid.

2. **Cool Slightly:** Allow the melted mixture to cool slightly but not solidify completely.

3. **Add Pumpkin Seed Oil and Cinnamon Essential Oil:** Once slightly cooled, stir in the pumpkin seed oil and cinnamon essential oil. Mix well to incorporate all ingredients.

4. **Blend Thoroughly:** Use a hand mixer or whisk to blend the ingredients thoroughly, ensuring a smooth and creamy consistency.

5. **Transfer to Jar:** Pour the body butter into a clean, airtight jar or container.

6. **Cool and Set:** Allow the body butter to cool and set at room temperature or in the refrigerator.

7. **Application:** After a bath or shower, apply a small amount of the body butter onto your skin, massaging gently for optimal absorption.

8. **Enjoy the Aroma:** Let the warm and inviting scent of cinnamon essential oil create a comforting atmosphere during application.

9. **Frequency:** Use this hydrating pumpkin seed oil and castor oil body butter regularly to keep your skin deeply moisturized, smooth, and pleasantly scented.

Nourishing Hazelnut Oil and Castor Oil Body Serum

Ingredients:

1. **Castor Oil (1/2 cup):** Castor oil provides deep moisturization, leaving your skin soft and hydrated.

2. **Hazelnut Oil (1/4 cup):** Hazelnut oil is rich in vitamins and fatty acids, offering nourishing benefits for the skin.

3. **Avocado Oil (1/4 cup):** Avocado oil is deeply hydrating and helps improve skin elasticity.

4. **Geranium Essential Oil (10 drops):** Geranium oil adds a floral aroma and is believed to have balancing effects on the skin.

Instructions:

1. **Combine Base Oils:** In a dark glass bottle, mix the castor oil, hazelnut oil, and avocado oil. These oils create a nourishing base for the body serum.

2. **Add Geranium Essential Oil:** Incorporate the drops of geranium essential oil into the mixture. Gently shake the bottle to ensure the oils are thoroughly blended.

3. **Patch Test:** Before applying the body serum to your skin, perform a patch test on a small area to ensure there are no

adverse reactions.

4. **Application:** Dispense a small amount of the body serum onto your palms and massage it onto your body, focusing on areas that need extra care.

5. **Use After Bath or Shower:** For best results, apply the body serum on damp skin after a bath or shower to lock in moisture.

6. **Enjoy the Fragrance:** Take a moment to enjoy the floral aroma of geranium essential oil as you apply the body serum.

7. **Frequency:** Use this nourishing hazelnut oil and castor oil body serum as part of your daily body care routine to promote skin hydration and a sense of balance.

This body serum combines the moisturizing benefits of castor oil, hazelnut oil, and avocado oil with the floral fragrance of geranium essential oil. Pamper your skin with this nutrient-rich blend to leave it feeling deeply nourished, hydrated, and delicately scented.

Rejuvenating Rosehip Oil and Castor Oil Body Elixir

Ingredients:

1. **Castor Oil (1/2 cup):** Castor oil provides deep moisturization, promoting soft and supple skin.

2. **Rosehip Oil (1/4 cup):** Rosehip oil is rich in antioxidants and essential fatty acids, offering rejuvenating benefits for the skin.

3. **Jojoba Oil (1/4 cup):** Jojoba oil closely resembles the skin's natural oils, providing additional hydration without a greasy feel.

4. **Rose Geranium Essential Oil (10 drops):** Rose geranium oil adds a floral and uplifting aroma while contributing to skin balance.

Instructions:

1. **Combine Base Oils:** In a dark glass bottle, mix the castor oil, rosehip oil, and jojoba oil. These oils create a nourishing base for the body elixir.

2. **Add Rose Geranium Essential Oil:** Incorporate the drops of rose geranium essential oil into the mixture. Gently shake the bottle to ensure the oils are thoroughly blended.

3. **Patch Test:** Before applying the body elixir to your skin, perform a patch test on a small area to ensure there are no adverse reactions.

4. **Application:** Dispense a small amount of the body elixir onto your palms and massage it onto your body, focusing on areas that need extra care.

5. **Use After Bath or Shower:** For best results, apply the body elixir on damp skin after a bath or shower to lock in moisture.

6. **Enjoy the Fragrance:** Take a moment to enjoy the floral and uplifting aroma of rose geranium essential oil as you apply the body elixir.

7. **Frequency:** Use this rejuvenating rosehip oil and castor oil body elixir as part of your daily body care routine to promote skin hydration and a sense of rejuvenation.

This body elixir combines the moisturizing benefits of castor oil, rosehip oil, and jojoba oil with the floral and uplifting fragrance of rose geranium essential oil. Pamper your skin with this luxurious blend to leave it feeling deeply nourished, hydrated, and delicately scented.

Soothing Sesame Oil and Castor Oil Body Balm

Ingredients:

1. **Castor Oil (1/2 cup):** Castor oil provides deep moisturization, leaving your skin soft and hydrated.

2. **Sesame Oil (1/4 cup):** Sesame oil is rich in vitamins and minerals, offering soothing benefits for the skin.

3. **Shea Butter (1/4 cup):** Shea butter is luxurious and contributes to intense hydration, promoting skin smoothness.

4. **Frankincense Essential Oil (10 drops):** Frankincense oil adds a warm and earthy fragrance while being believed to have skin-soothing properties.

Instructions:

1. **Melt Shea Butter and Oils:** In a double boiler or a heat-safe bowl over simmering water, melt the shea butter and castor oil until they form a liquid.

2. **Cool Slightly:** Allow the melted mixture to cool slightly but not solidify completely.

3. **Add Sesame Oil and Frankincense Essential Oil:** Once slightly cooled, stir in the sesame oil and frankincense essential oil. Mix well to incorporate all ingredients.

4. **Blend Thoroughly:** Use a hand mixer or whisk to blend the ingredients thoroughly, ensuring a smooth and creamy consistency.

5. **Transfer to Jar:** Pour the body balm into a clean, airtight jar or container.

6. **Cool and Set:** Allow the body balm to cool and set at room temperature or in the refrigerator.

7. **Application:** After a bath or shower, apply a small amount of the body balm onto your skin, massaging gently for optimal absorption.

8. **Enjoy the Aroma:** Let the warm and earthy scent of frankincense essential oil create a soothing atmosphere during application.

9. **Frequency:** Use this soothing sesame oil and castor oil body balm regularly to keep your skin deeply moisturized, smooth, and pleasantly scented.

Invigorating Pine Essential Oil and Castor Oil Body Scrub

Ingredients:

1. **Castor Oil (1/2 cup):** Castor oil provides deep moisturization, promoting soft and supple skin.

2. **Jojoba Oil (1/4 cup):** Jojoba oil closely resembles the skin's natural oils, offering additional hydration without a greasy feel.

3. **Granulated Sugar (1/2 cup):** Granulated sugar provides gentle exfoliation, removing dead skin cells for a smoother complexion.

4. **Pine Essential Oil (15 drops):** Pine oil has an invigorating and refreshing fragrance, promoting a sense of vitality.

Instructions:

1. **Combine Base Oils:** In a mixing bowl, blend the castor oil and jojoba oil. These oils create a moisturizing base for the body scrub.

2. **Add Pine Essential Oil:** Incorporate the drops of pine essential oil into the oil mixture. Stir well to ensure an even distribution of the fragrance.

3. **Integrate Sugar:** Gradually add the granulated sugar to the oil and essential oil mixture. Stir until the sugar is evenly coated with the oils.

4. **Test Consistency:** Adjust the sugar and oil proportions if needed until you achieve a scrub with a thick, spreadable consistency.

5. **Transfer to Container:** Pour the body scrub into a clean, airtight jar or container.

6. **Cool and Set:** Allow the body scrub to cool and set at room temperature.

7. **Application:** In the shower, take a small amount of the body scrub and massage it onto damp skin in gentle circular motions. Focus on areas that need revitalization.

8. **Rinse Off:** Rinse off the scrub thoroughly with warm water, leaving your skin feeling refreshed.

9. **Pat Dry:** Gently pat your skin dry with a towel. Avoid rubbing too vigorously to allow the oils to remain on your skin.

10. **Enjoy the Aroma:** Let the invigorating scent of pine essential oil awaken your senses and create a refreshing atmosphere.

11. **Frequency:** Use this invigorating pine essential oil and castor oil body scrub a few times a week to rejuvenate your skin and elevate your senses.

Soothing Neem Oil and Castor Oil Body Butter

Ingredients:

1. **Castor Oil (1/2 cup):** Castor oil provides deep moisturization, promoting soft and supple skin.

2. **Neem Oil (1/4 cup):** Neem oil is known for its soothing and nourishing properties, offering benefits for the skin.

3. **Cocoa Butter (1/4 cup):** Cocoa butter adds a luxurious feel and enhances the overall moisturizing properties of the body butter.

4. **Lavender Essential Oil (10 drops):** Lavender oil adds a calming fragrance and complements the soothing effects of neem oil.

Instructions:

1. **Melt Cocoa Butter and Oils:** In a double boiler or a heat-safe bowl over simmering water, melt the cocoa butter and castor oil until they form a liquid.

2. **Cool Slightly:** Allow the melted mixture to cool slightly but not solidify completely.

3. **Add Neem Oil and Lavender Essential Oil:** Once slightly cooled, stir in the neem oil and lavender essential oil. Mix well

to incorporate all ingredients.

4. **Blend Thoroughly:** Use a hand mixer or whisk to blend the ingredients thoroughly, ensuring a smooth and creamy consistency.

5. **Transfer to Jar:** Pour the body butter into a clean, airtight jar or container.

6. **Cool and Set:** Allow the body butter to cool and set at room temperature or in the refrigerator.

7. **Application:** After a bath or shower, apply a small amount of the body butter onto your skin, massaging gently for optimal absorption.

8. **Enjoy the Aroma:** Let the calming scent of lavender essential oil create a soothing atmosphere during application.

9. **Frequency:** Use this soothing neem oil and castor oil body butter regularly to keep your skin deeply moisturized, smooth, and pleasantly scented.

Revitalizing Rosemary Oil and Castor Oil Body Scrub

Ingredients:

1. **Castor Oil (1/2 cup):** Castor oil provides deep moisturization, promoting soft and supple skin.

2. **Coconut Oil (1/4 cup):** Coconut oil adds a light texture and enhances the overall nourishing properties of the body scrub.

3. **Brown Sugar (1/2 cup):** Brown sugar provides gentle exfoliation, removing dead skin cells for a smoother complexion.

4. **Rosemary Essential Oil (15 drops):** Rosemary oil has a invigorating and herbaceous fragrance, promoting a sense of revitalization.

Instructions:

1. **Melt Coconut Oil:** In a microwave-safe bowl, melt the coconut oil until it becomes a liquid.

2. **Combine Ingredients:** In a mixing bowl, combine the melted coconut oil, castor oil, brown sugar, and rosemary essential oil. Mix well until you achieve a consistent scrub.

3. **Test Consistency:** Adjust the sugar and oil proportions if needed until you achieve a scrub with a thick, spreadable

consistency.

4. **Transfer to Container:** Pour the body scrub into a clean, airtight jar or container.

5. **Cool and Set:** Allow the body scrub to cool and set at room temperature.

6. **Application:** In the shower, take a small amount of the body scrub and massage it onto damp skin in gentle circular motions. Focus on areas that need revitalization.

7. **Rinse Off:** Rinse off the scrub thoroughly with warm water, leaving your skin feeling refreshed.

8. **Pat Dry:** Gently pat your skin dry with a towel. Avoid rubbing too vigorously to allow the oils to remain on your skin.

9. **Enjoy the Aroma:** Let the invigorating scent of rosemary essential oil awaken your senses and create a revitalizing atmosphere.

10. **Frequency:** Use this revitalizing rosemary oil and castor oil body scrub a few times a week to rejuvenate your skin and uplift your senses.

Uplifting Lemon Balm Essential Oil and Castor Oil Body Lotion

Ingredients:

1. **Castor Oil (1/2 cup):** Castor oil provides deep moisturization, promoting soft and supple skin.

2. **Sweet Almond Oil (1/4 cup):** Sweet almond oil is lightweight and easily absorbed, contributing to overall skin hydration.

3. **Shea Butter (1/4 cup):** Shea butter adds a luxurious feel and enhances the overall moisturizing properties of the body lotion.

4. **Lemon Balm Essential Oil (15 drops):** Lemon balm oil has a refreshing and uplifting fragrance, promoting a sense of positivity.

Instructions:

1. **Melt Shea Butter and Oils:** In a double boiler or a heat-safe bowl over simmering water, melt the shea butter and castor oil until they form a liquid.

2. **Cool Slightly:** Allow the melted mixture to cool slightly but not solidify completely.

3. **Add Sweet Almond Oil and Lemon Balm Essential Oil:** Once slightly cooled, stir in the sweet almond oil and lemon balm essential oil. Mix well to incorporate all ingredients.

4. **Blend Thoroughly:** Use a hand mixer or whisk to blend the ingredients thoroughly, ensuring a smooth and creamy consistency.

5. **Transfer to Jar:** Pour the body lotion into a clean, airtight jar or container.

6. **Cool and Set:** Allow the body lotion to cool and set at room temperature or in the refrigerator.

7. **Application:** After a bath or shower, apply a generous amount of the body lotion onto your body, focusing on areas that need extra care.

8. **Enjoy the Aroma:** Let the refreshing scent of lemon balm essential oil uplift your spirits and create a positive atmosphere.

9. **Frequency:** Use this uplifting lemon balm essential oil and castor oil body lotion daily to keep your skin deeply moisturized and enjoy the positive effects on your mood.

Revitalizing Orange Oil and Castor Oil Body Scrub for Morning Energization

Ingredients:

1. **Castor Oil (1/2 cup):** Castor oil provides deep moisturization, leaving your skin soft and hydrated.

2. **Coconut Oil (1/4 cup):** Coconut oil adds a light texture and enhances the overall nourishing properties of the body scrub.

3. **Granulated Sugar (1/2 cup):** Granulated sugar provides gentle exfoliation, removing dead skin cells for a smoother complexion.

4. **Orange Essential Oil (15 drops):** Orange oil has a refreshing and invigorating fragrance, revitalizing the senses in the morning.

Instructions:

1. **Melt Coconut Oil:** In a microwave-safe bowl, melt the coconut oil until it becomes a liquid.

2. **Combine Ingredients:** In a mixing bowl, combine the melted coconut oil, castor oil, granulated sugar, and orange essential oil. Mix well until you achieve a consistent scrub.

3. **Test Consistency:** Adjust the sugar and oil proportions if needed until you achieve a scrub with a thick, spreadable consistency.

4. **Transfer to Container:** Pour the body scrub into a clean, airtight jar or container.

5. **Cool and Set:** Allow the body scrub to cool and set at room temperature.

6. **Application:** In the morning, take a small amount of the body scrub and massage it onto damp skin in gentle circular motions. Focus on areas that need revitalization.

7. **Rinse Off:** Rinse off the scrub thoroughly with warm water, leaving your skin feeling refreshed.

8. **Pat Dry:** Gently pat your skin dry with a towel. Avoid rubbing too vigorously to allow the oils to remain on your skin.

9. **Enjoy the Aroma:** Allow the invigorating scent of orange essential oil to awaken your senses and prepare you for the day ahead.

10. **Frequency:** Use this revitalizing orange oil and castor oil body scrub a few times a week in the morning to start your day with refreshed and energized skin.

Soothing Oat Milk and Castor Oil Body Lotion

Ingredients:

1. **Castor Oil (1/2 cup):** Castor oil provides deep moisturization, promoting soft and supple skin.

2. **Oat Milk (1/4 cup):** Oat milk is soothing and nourishing, known for its calming effects on the skin.

3. **Shea Butter (1/4 cup):** Shea butter is rich in fatty acids and vitamins, contributing to intense hydration and nourishment.

4. **Vanilla Extract (1 teaspoon):** Vanilla extract adds a sweet aroma, enhancing the overall sensory experience.

Instructions:

1. **Melt Shea Butter and Oils:** In a double boiler or a heat-safe bowl over simmering water, melt the shea butter and castor oil until they form a liquid.

2. **Cool Slightly:** Allow the melted mixture to cool slightly but not solidify completely.

3. **Add Oat Milk and Vanilla Extract:** Once slightly cooled, stir in the oat milk and vanilla extract. Mix well to incorporate all ingredients.

4. **Blend Thoroughly:** Use a hand mixer or whisk to blend the ingredients thoroughly, ensuring a smooth and creamy consistency.

5. **Transfer to Jar:** Pour the body lotion into a clean, airtight jar or container.

6. **Cool and Set:** Allow the body lotion to cool and set at room temperature or in the refrigerator.

7. **Application:** After a bath or shower, apply a generous amount of the body lotion onto your body, focusing on areas that need extra care.

8. **Enjoy the Aroma:** Let the sweet scent of vanilla and the soothing properties of oat milk envelop your senses.

9. **Frequency:** Use this soothing oat milk and castor oil body lotion daily to keep your skin deeply moisturized, soft, and delicately scented.

Nourishing Evening Primrose and Castor Oil Body Oil

Ingredients:

1. **Castor Oil (1/2 cup):** Castor oil provides deep moisturization, promoting soft and supple skin.

2. **Evening Primrose Oil (1/4 cup):** Evening primrose oil is rich in gamma-linolenic acid, known for its nourishing and skin-soothing properties.

3. **Jojoba Oil (1/4 cup):** Jojoba oil closely resembles the skin's natural oils, offering additional hydration without a greasy feel.

4. **Lavender Essential Oil (10 drops):** Lavender oil adds a calming fragrance and complements the overall soothing effects of evening primrose oil.

Instructions:

1. **Combine Base Oils:** In a dark glass bottle, mix the castor oil, evening primrose oil, and jojoba oil. These oils create a nourishing base for the body oil.

2. **Add Lavender Essential Oil:** Incorporate the drops of lavender essential oil into the mixture. Gently shake the bottle to ensure the oils are thoroughly blended.

3. **Patch Test:** Before applying the body oil to your skin, perform a patch test on a small area to ensure there are no adverse reactions.

4. **Application:** Dispense a small amount of the body oil onto your palms and massage it onto your body, focusing on areas that need extra care.

5. **Use After Bath or Shower:** For best results, apply the body oil on damp skin after a bath or shower to lock in moisture.

6. **Enjoy the Fragrance:** Take a moment to enjoy the calming aroma of lavender essential oil as you apply the body oil.

7. **Frequency:** Use this nourishing evening primrose and castor oil body oil as part of your daily body care routine to promote skin hydration and a sense of tranquility.

This body oil combines the moisturizing benefits of castor oil, evening primrose oil, and jojoba oil with the calming properties of lavender essential oil. Pamper your skin with this aromatic blend to leave it feeling deeply nourished, hydrated, and delicately scented.

Hydrating Pumpkin Seed Oil and Castor Oil Body Butter

Ingredients:

1. **Castor Oil (1/2 cup):** Castor oil provides deep moisturization, leaving your skin soft and hydrated.

2. **Pumpkin Seed Oil (1/4 cup):** Pumpkin seed oil is rich in antioxidants and essential fatty acids, offering nourishing benefits for the skin.

3. **Cocoa Butter (1/4 cup):** Cocoa butter adds a luxurious feel and enhances the overall moisturizing properties of the body butter.

4. **Cinnamon Essential Oil (10 drops):** Cinnamon oil adds a warm and inviting fragrance while promoting a sense of comfort.

Instructions:

1. **Melt Cocoa Butter and Oils:** In a double boiler or a heat-safe bowl over simmering water, melt the cocoa butter and castor oil until they form a liquid.

2. **Cool Slightly:** Allow the melted mixture to cool slightly but not solidify completely.

3. **Add Pumpkin Seed Oil and Cinnamon Essential Oil:** Once slightly cooled, stir in the pumpkin seed oil and cinnamon essential oil. Mix well to incorporate all ingredients.

4. **Blend Thoroughly:** Use a hand mixer or whisk to blend the ingredients thoroughly, ensuring a smooth and creamy consistency.

5. **Transfer to Jar:** Pour the body butter into a clean, airtight jar or container.

6. **Cool and Set:** Allow the body butter to cool and set at room temperature or in the refrigerator.

7. **Application:** After a bath or shower, apply a small amount of the body butter onto your skin, massaging gently for optimal absorption.

8. **Enjoy the Aroma:** Let the warm and inviting scent of cinnamon essential oil create a comforting atmosphere during application.

9. **Frequency:** Use this hydrating pumpkin seed oil and castor oil body butter regularly to keep your skin deeply moisturized, smooth, and pleasantly scented.

Nourishing Hazelnut Oil and Castor Oil Body Serum

Ingredients:

1. **Castor Oil (1/2 cup):** Castor oil provides deep moisturization, leaving your skin soft and hydrated.

2. **Hazelnut Oil (1/4 cup):** Hazelnut oil is rich in vitamins and fatty acids, offering nourishing benefits for the skin.

3. **Avocado Oil (1/4 cup):** Avocado oil is deeply hydrating and helps improve skin elasticity.

4. **Geranium Essential Oil (10 drops):** Geranium oil adds a floral aroma and is believed to have balancing effects on the skin.

Instructions:

1. **Combine Base Oils:** In a dark glass bottle, mix the castor oil, hazelnut oil, and avocado oil. These oils create a nourishing base for the body serum.

2. **Add Geranium Essential Oil:** Incorporate the drops of geranium essential oil into the mixture. Gently shake the bottle to ensure the oils are thoroughly blended.

3. **Patch Test:** Before applying the body serum to your skin, perform a patch test on a small area to ensure there are no

adverse reactions.

4. **Application:** Dispense a small amount of the body serum onto your palms and massage it onto your body, focusing on areas that need extra care.

5. **Use After Bath or Shower:** For best results, apply the body serum on damp skin after a bath or shower to lock in moisture.

6. **Enjoy the Fragrance:** Take a moment to enjoy the floral aroma of geranium essential oil as you apply the body serum.

7. **Frequency:** Use this nourishing hazelnut oil and castor oil body serum as part of your daily body care routine to promote skin hydration and a sense of balance.

This body serum combines the moisturizing benefits of castor oil, hazelnut oil, and avocado oil with the floral fragrance of geranium essential oil. Pamper your skin with this nutrient-rich blend to leave it feeling deeply nourished, hydrated, and delicately scented.

Rejuvenating Rosehip Oil and Castor Oil Body Elixir

Ingredients:

1. **Castor Oil (1/2 cup):** Castor oil provides deep moisturization, promoting soft and supple skin.

2. **Rosehip Oil (1/4 cup):** Rosehip oil is rich in antioxidants and essential fatty acids, offering rejuvenating benefits for the skin.

3. **Jojoba Oil (1/4 cup):** Jojoba oil closely resembles the skin's natural oils, providing additional hydration without a greasy feel.

4. **Rose Geranium Essential Oil (10 drops):** Rose geranium oil adds a floral and uplifting aroma while contributing to skin balance.

Instructions:

1. **Combine Base Oils:** In a dark glass bottle, mix the castor oil, rosehip oil, and jojoba oil. These oils create a nourishing base for the body elixir.

2. **Add Rose Geranium Essential Oil:** Incorporate the drops of rose geranium essential oil into the mixture. Gently shake the bottle to ensure the oils are thoroughly blended.

3. **Patch Test:** Before applying the body elixir to your skin, perform a patch test on a small area to ensure there are no adverse reactions.

4. **Application:** Dispense a small amount of the body elixir onto your palms and massage it onto your body, focusing on areas that need extra care.

5. **Use After Bath or Shower:** For best results, apply the body elixir on damp skin after a bath or shower to lock in moisture.

6. **Enjoy the Fragrance:** Take a moment to enjoy the floral and uplifting aroma of rose geranium essential oil as you apply the body elixir.

7. **Frequency:** Use this rejuvenating rosehip oil and castor oil body elixir as part of your daily body care routine to promote skin hydration and a sense of rejuvenation.

This body elixir combines the moisturizing benefits of castor oil, rosehip oil, and jojoba oil with the floral and uplifting fragrance of rose geranium essential oil. Pamper your skin with this luxurious blend to leave it feeling deeply nourished, hydrated, and delicately scented.

Soothing Sesame Oil and Castor Oil Body Balm

Ingredients:

1. **Castor Oil (1/2 cup):** Castor oil provides deep moisturization, leaving your skin soft and hydrated.

2. **Sesame Oil (1/4 cup):** Sesame oil is rich in vitamins and minerals, offering soothing benefits for the skin.

3. **Shea Butter (1/4 cup):** Shea butter is luxurious and contributes to intense hydration, promoting skin smoothness.

4. **Frankincense Essential Oil (10 drops):** Frankincense oil adds a warm and earthy fragrance while being believed to have skin-soothing properties.

Instructions:

1. **Melt Shea Butter and Oils:** In a double boiler or a heat-safe bowl over simmering water, melt the shea butter and castor oil until they form a liquid.

2. **Cool Slightly:** Allow the melted mixture to cool slightly but not solidify completely.

3. **Add Sesame Oil and Frankincense Essential Oil:** Once slightly cooled, stir in the sesame oil and frankincense essential oil. Mix well to incorporate all ingredients.

4. **Blend Thoroughly:** Use a hand mixer or whisk to blend the ingredients thoroughly, ensuring a smooth and creamy consistency.

5. **Transfer to Jar:** Pour the body balm into a clean, airtight jar or container.

6. **Cool and Set:** Allow the body balm to cool and set at room temperature or in the refrigerator.

7. **Application:** After a bath or shower, apply a small amount of the body balm onto your skin, massaging gently for optimal absorption.

8. **Enjoy the Aroma:** Let the warm and earthy scent of frankincense essential oil create a soothing atmosphere during application.

9. **Frequency:** Use this soothing sesame oil and castor oil body balm regularly to keep your skin deeply moisturized, smooth, and pleasantly scented.

Invigorating Pine Essential Oil and Castor Oil Body Scrub

Ingredients:

1. **Castor Oil (1/2 cup):** Castor oil provides deep moisturization, promoting soft and supple skin.

2. **Jojoba Oil (1/4 cup):** Jojoba oil closely resembles the skin's natural oils, offering additional hydration without a greasy feel.

3. **Granulated Sugar (1/2 cup):** Granulated sugar provides gentle exfoliation, removing dead skin cells for a smoother complexion.

4. **Pine Essential Oil (15 drops):** Pine oil has an invigorating and refreshing fragrance, promoting a sense of vitality.

Instructions:

1. **Combine Base Oils:** In a mixing bowl, blend the castor oil and jojoba oil. These oils create a moisturizing base for the body scrub.

2. **Add Pine Essential Oil:** Incorporate the drops of pine essential oil into the oil mixture. Stir well to ensure an even distribution of the fragrance.

3. **Integrate Sugar:** Gradually add the granulated sugar to the oil and essential oil mixture. Stir until the sugar is evenly coated with the oils.

4. **Test Consistency:** Adjust the sugar and oil proportions if needed until you achieve a scrub with a thick, spreadable consistency.

5. **Transfer to Container:** Pour the body scrub into a clean, airtight jar or container.

6. **Cool and Set:** Allow the body scrub to cool and set at room temperature.

7. **Application:** In the shower, take a small amount of the body scrub and massage it onto damp skin in gentle circular motions. Focus on areas that need revitalization.

8. **Rinse Off:** Rinse off the scrub thoroughly with warm water, leaving your skin feeling refreshed.

9. **Pat Dry:** Gently pat your skin dry with a towel. Avoid rubbing too vigorously to allow the oils to remain on your skin.

10. **Enjoy the Aroma:** Let the invigorating scent of pine essential oil awaken your senses and create a refreshing atmosphere.

11. **Frequency:** Use this invigorating pine essential oil and castor oil body scrub a few times a week to rejuvenate your skin and elevate your senses.

Soothing Neem Oil and Castor Oil Body Butter

Ingredients:

1. **Castor Oil (1/2 cup):** Castor oil provides deep moisturization, promoting soft and supple skin.

2. **Neem Oil (1/4 cup):** Neem oil is known for its soothing and nourishing properties, offering benefits for the skin.

3. **Cocoa Butter (1/4 cup):** Cocoa butter adds a luxurious feel and enhances the overall moisturizing properties of the body butter.

4. **Lavender Essential Oil (10 drops):** Lavender oil adds a calming fragrance and complements the soothing effects of neem oil.

Instructions:

1. **Melt Cocoa Butter and Oils:** In a double boiler or a heat-safe bowl over simmering water, melt the cocoa butter and castor oil until they form a liquid.

2. **Cool Slightly:** Allow the melted mixture to cool slightly but not solidify completely.

3. **Add Neem Oil and Lavender Essential Oil:** Once slightly cooled, stir in the neem oil and lavender essential oil. Mix well

to incorporate all ingredients.

4. **Blend Thoroughly:** Use a hand mixer or whisk to blend the ingredients thoroughly, ensuring a smooth and creamy consistency.

5. **Transfer to Jar:** Pour the body butter into a clean, airtight jar or container.

6. **Cool and Set:** Allow the body butter to cool and set at room temperature or in the refrigerator.

7. **Application:** After a bath or shower, apply a small amount of the body butter onto your skin, massaging gently for optimal absorption.

8. **Enjoy the Aroma:** Let the calming scent of lavender essential oil create a soothing atmosphere during application.

9. **Frequency:** Use this soothing neem oil and castor oil body butter regularly to keep your skin deeply moisturized, smooth, and pleasantly scented.

Revitalizing Rosemary Oil and Castor Oil Body Scrub

Ingredients:

1. **Castor Oil (1/2 cup):** Castor oil provides deep moisturization, promoting soft and supple skin.

2. **Coconut Oil (1/4 cup):** Coconut oil adds a light texture and enhances the overall nourishing properties of the body scrub.

3. **Brown Sugar (1/2 cup):** Brown sugar provides gentle exfoliation, removing dead skin cells for a smoother complexion.

4. **Rosemary Essential Oil (15 drops):** Rosemary oil has a invigorating and herbaceous fragrance, promoting a sense of revitalization.

Instructions:

1. **Melt Coconut Oil:** In a microwave-safe bowl, melt the coconut oil until it becomes a liquid.

2. **Combine Ingredients:** In a mixing bowl, combine the melted coconut oil, castor oil, brown sugar, and rosemary essential oil. Mix well until you achieve a consistent scrub.

3. **Test Consistency:** Adjust the sugar and oil proportions if needed until you achieve a scrub with a thick, spreadable

consistency.

4. **Transfer to Container:** Pour the body scrub into a clean, airtight jar or container.

5. **Cool and Set:** Allow the body scrub to cool and set at room temperature.

6. **Application:** In the shower, take a small amount of the body scrub and massage it onto damp skin in gentle circular motions. Focus on areas that need revitalization.

7. **Rinse Off:** Rinse off the scrub thoroughly with warm water, leaving your skin feeling refreshed.

8. **Pat Dry:** Gently pat your skin dry with a towel. Avoid rubbing too vigorously to allow the oils to remain on your skin.

9. **Enjoy the Aroma:** Let the invigorating scent of rosemary essential oil awaken your senses and create a revitalizing atmosphere.

10. **Frequency:** Use this revitalizing rosemary oil and castor oil body scrub a few times a week to rejuvenate your skin and uplift your senses.

Uplifting Lemon Balm Essential Oil and Castor Oil Body Lotion

Ingredients:

1. **Castor Oil (1/2 cup):** Castor oil provides deep moisturization, promoting soft and supple skin.

2. **Sweet Almond Oil (1/4 cup):** Sweet almond oil is lightweight and easily absorbed, contributing to overall skin hydration.

3. **Shea Butter (1/4 cup):** Shea butter adds a luxurious feel and enhances the overall moisturizing properties of the body lotion.

4. **Lemon Balm Essential Oil (15 drops):** Lemon balm oil has a refreshing and uplifting fragrance, promoting a sense of positivity.

Instructions:

1. **Melt Shea Butter and Oils:** In a double boiler or a heat-safe bowl over simmering water, melt the shea butter and castor oil until they form a liquid.

2. **Cool Slightly:** Allow the melted mixture to cool slightly but not solidify completely.

3. **Add Sweet Almond Oil and Lemon Balm Essential Oil:** Once slightly cooled, stir in the sweet almond oil and lemon balm essential oil. Mix well to incorporate all ingredients.

4. **Blend Thoroughly:** Use a hand mixer or whisk to blend the ingredients thoroughly, ensuring a smooth and creamy consistency.

5. **Transfer to Jar:** Pour the body lotion into a clean, airtight jar or container.

6. **Cool and Set:** Allow the body lotion to cool and set at room temperature or in the refrigerator.

7. **Application:** After a bath or shower, apply a generous amount of the body lotion onto your body, focusing on areas that need extra care.

8. **Enjoy the Aroma:** Let the refreshing scent of lemon balm essential oil uplift your spirits and create a positive atmosphere.

9. **Frequency:** Use this uplifting lemon balm essential oil and castor oil body lotion daily to keep your skin deeply moisturized and enjoy the positive effects on your mood.

CHAPTER ELEVEN

Hair Care Recipes

Castor oil, a versatile elixir, acts as a natural conditioner, promoting hydration and strengthening hair follicles. As we delve into the enchanting world of these castor oil concoctions, you'll find yourself immersed in the luxurious scents of essential oils and the wholesome embrace of natural ingredients. Each recipe is a testament to the belief that self-care is an art, and your hair deserves nothing short of the finest ingredients nature has to offer. Whether you're on a quest for voluminous tresses, a soothing scalp treatment, or a remedy for damaged ends, let this chapter be your guide. Transform your haircare routine into a ritual of self-love, and let the alchemy of castor oil breathe new life into your locks. Get ready to witness the magic as your hair becomes a testament to the natural wonders found within the pages of this chapter.

CHAPTER TWELVE

Recipes for Oily Hair

Revitalizing Citrus-Castor Exfoliating Scrub

Ingredients:

1. **Castor Oil (1 tablespoon):** The base of this scrub, castor oil, adds hydration while promoting gentle exfoliation.

2. **Fine Sugar (2 tablespoons):** Sugar serves as a natural exfoliant, helping to remove dead skin cells and reveal a brighter complexion.

3. **Lemon Juice (1 tablespoon):** Packed with vitamin C, lemon juice helps lighten dark spots, promoting an even skin tone.

4. **Sweet Orange Essential Oil (5 drops):** The uplifting aroma of sweet orange essential oil adds a refreshing and invigorating element to the scrub.

5. **Vanilla Extract (1/2 teaspoon):** Vanilla not only provides a delightful scent but also contains antioxidants that can soothe and calm the skin.

Instructions:

1. **Combine the Ingredients:** In a bowl, mix the castor oil, fine sugar, lemon juice, sweet orange essential oil, and vanilla extract. Stir well until the ingredients form a cohesive scrub.

2. **Patch Test:** Prior to applying the scrub to your face, perform a patch test on a small area of skin to ensure compatibility, especially if you have sensitive skin.

3. **Application:** Gently massage the scrub onto your clean, damp face using circular motions. Focus on areas that may need extra exfoliation, such as the nose and forehead.

4. **Allow to Sit:** Let the scrub sit on your skin for a few minutes to allow the beneficial properties of the ingredients to work their magic.

5. **Rinse Off:** Rinse your face with lukewarm water, making sure to remove all traces of the scrub. Pat your face dry with a clean towel.

6. **Follow with Moisturizer:** Finish your skincare routine by applying your favorite moisturizer to keep your skin hydrated

after the exfoliation.

7. **Frequency:** Use this revitalizing citrus-castor exfoliating scrub once or twice a week to maintain smooth and rejuvenated skin.

Balancing Castor Oil and Black Seed Oil Hair Mask for Oily Hair

Ingredients:

1. **Castor Oil (2 tablespoons):** Castor oil helps to moisturize the hair and scalp while regulating oil production.

2. **Black Seed Oil (1 tablespoon):** Black seed oil has antimicrobial properties and helps balance oil production on the scalp.

3. **Apple Cider Vinegar (1 tablespoon):** Apple cider vinegar helps to remove excess oil, product buildup, and restores the pH balance of the scalp.

4. **Lemon Juice (1 tablespoon):** Lemon juice helps control oil and adds a refreshing scent.

5. **Aloe Vera Gel (1 tablespoon):** Aloe vera soothes the scalp, balances oil, and promotes overall scalp health.

Instructions:

1. **Mixing the Ingredients:** In a bowl, combine castor oil, black seed oil, apple cider vinegar, lemon juice, and aloe vera gel. Mix well until you achieve a smooth consistency.

2. **Application:** Part your hair into sections and apply the mix-

ture to your scalp and hair, focusing on the roots. Use a brush or your fingertips to evenly distribute the mask.

3. **Massage:** Gently massage the mask into your scalp using circular motions. This stimulates blood circulation and ensures even distribution.

4. **Hair Length:** If you have oily hair, focus more on the roots and the mid-lengths of your hair. Avoid applying too much on the ends.

5. **Leave-In:** Leave the mask in for about 30 minutes to allow the ingredients to work on your scalp and hair. You can cover your hair with a shower cap for better absorption.

6. **Rinse:** Rinse your hair thoroughly with lukewarm water. You may use a mild sulfate-free shampoo if needed.

7. **Condition (Optional):** Depending on your hair type, you can follow up with a light conditioner, but avoid applying it to the scalp.

8. **Frequency:** Use this mask once a week or as needed to help balance oil production and maintain a healthy scalp.

Clarifying Castor Oil and Jojoba Oil Hair Mask for Oily Hair

Ingredients:

1. **Castor Oil (2 tablespoons):** Castor oil helps control excess oil production on the scalp.

2. **Jojoba Oil (1 tablespoon):** Jojoba oil mimics the natural oils of the scalp, providing balance without promoting excess oiliness.

3. **Lemon Juice (2 tablespoons):** Lemon juice helps cut through excess oil and adds a refreshing scent.

4. **Tea Tree Essential Oil (5 drops):** Tea tree oil has antimicrobial properties that help combat oiliness and maintain a healthy scalp.

5. **Aloe Vera Gel (1 tablespoon):** Aloe vera soothes the scalp and provides hydration without adding heaviness.

Instructions:

1. **Mixing the Ingredients:** In a bowl, combine castor oil, jojoba oil, lemon juice, tea tree essential oil, and aloe vera gel. Stir well to ensure all ingredients are thoroughly mixed.

2. **Application:** Part your hair into sections and apply the mix-

ture to your scalp and hair, focusing on the roots. Use a brush or your fingertips to evenly distribute the mask.

3. **Massage:** Gently massage the mask into your scalp using circular motions. This helps stimulate blood circulation and ensures even application.

4. **Hair Length:** Focus the application on the roots and the mid-lengths of your hair. Avoid applying too much on the ends, especially if they tend to be drier.

5. **Leave-In:** Leave the mask on for about 20-30 minutes. You can cover your hair with a shower cap for better absorption.

6. **Rinse:** Rinse your hair thoroughly with lukewarm water. You may use a mild sulfate-free shampoo if needed.

7. **Condition (Optional):** Depending on your hair type, you can follow up with a light conditioner, but avoid applying it to the scalp.

8. **Frequency:** Use this mask once a week or as needed to help control oiliness and maintain a healthy scalp.

Purifying Castor Oil and Juniper Oil Hair Mask for Oily Hair

Ingredients:

1. **Castor Oil (2 tablespoons):** Castor oil helps control excess oil production on the scalp.

2. **Jojoba Oil (1 tablespoon):** Jojoba oil balances oiliness without adding additional weight to the hair.

3. **Juniper Essential Oil (7 drops):** Juniper oil has astringent properties that help purify the scalp and regulate oil production.

4. **Lemon Juice (1 tablespoon):** Lemon juice cuts through excess oil and adds a refreshing scent.

5. **Aloe Vera Gel (1 tablespoon):** Aloe vera soothes the scalp and provides hydration without making the hair greasy.

Instructions:

1. **Mixing the Ingredients:** In a bowl, combine castor oil, jojoba oil, juniper essential oil, lemon juice, and aloe vera gel. Stir well to ensure all ingredients are thoroughly mixed.

2. **Application:** Part your hair into sections and apply the mixture to your scalp and hair, focusing on the roots. Use a brush

or your fingertips to evenly distribute the mask.

3. **Massage:** Gently massage the mask into your scalp using circular motions. This helps stimulate blood circulation and ensures even application.

4. **Hair Length:** Focus the application on the roots and the mid-lengths of your hair. Avoid applying too much on the ends.

5. **Leave-In:** Leave the mask on for about 20-30 minutes. You can cover your hair with a shower cap for better absorption.

6. **Rinse:** Rinse your hair thoroughly with lukewarm water. You may use a mild sulfate-free shampoo if needed.

7. **Condition (Optional):** Depending on your hair type, you can follow up with a light conditioner, but avoid applying it to the scalp.

8. **Frequency:** Use this mask once a week or as needed to help purify the scalp, control oiliness, and maintain a healthy balance.

Balancing Castor Oil and Tea Tree Oil Scalp Treatment for Oily Hair

Ingredients:

1. **Castor Oil (2 tablespoons):** Castor oil helps control excess oil production on the scalp.

2. **Jojoba Oil (1 tablespoon):** Jojoba oil balances oiliness without making the hair greasy.

3. **Tea Tree Essential Oil (8 drops):** Tea tree oil has antimicrobial properties that help combat oiliness and maintain scalp health.

4. **Lemon Juice (1 tablespoon):** Lemon juice helps cut through excess oil and adds a refreshing scent.

5. **Aloe Vera Gel (1 tablespoon):** Aloe vera soothes the scalp and provides hydration without making the hair heavy.

Instructions:

1. **Mixing the Ingredients:** In a bowl, combine castor oil, jojoba oil, tea tree essential oil, lemon juice, and aloe vera gel. Stir well to ensure all ingredients are thoroughly mixed.

2. **Application:** Section your hair and apply the mixture to your scalp and roots, focusing on areas prone to oiliness. Use a brush or your fingertips to evenly distribute the treatment.

3. **Massage:** Gently massage the scalp in circular motions to

stimulate blood circulation and ensure even absorption.

4. **Leave-In:** Leave the treatment on for about 20-30 minutes. You can cover your hair with a shower cap for better penetration.

5. **Rinse:** Rinse your hair thoroughly with lukewarm water. You may use a mild sulfate-free shampoo if needed.

6. **Condition (Optional):** Depending on your hair type, you can follow up with a light conditioner, but avoid applying it to the scalp.

7. **Frequency:** Use this treatment once a week or as needed to help balance oil production and maintain a healthy scalp.

Revitalizing Castor Oil and Rosemary Essential Oil Scalp Treatment for Oily Hair

Ingredients:

1. **Castor Oil (2 tablespoons):** Castor oil helps control excess oil production on the scalp.

2. **Grapeseed Oil (1 tablespoon):** Grapeseed oil is lightweight and helps balance oiliness without weighing down the hair.

3. **Rosemary Essential Oil (8 drops):** Rosemary oil promotes scalp health, regulates oil production, and adds a refreshing fragrance.

4. **Lemon Juice (1 tablespoon):** Lemon juice cuts through excess oil and adds a revitalizing scent.

5. **Aloe Vera Gel (1 tablespoon):** Aloe vera soothes the scalp, provides hydration, and maintains a healthy balance.

Instructions:

1. **Mixing the Ingredients:** In a bowl, combine castor oil, grapeseed oil, rosemary essential oil, lemon juice, and aloe vera gel. Stir well to ensure all ingredients are thoroughly mixed.

2. **Application:** Section your hair and apply the mixture to

your scalp and roots, focusing on areas prone to oiliness. Use a brush or your fingertips to evenly distribute the treatment.

3. **Massage:** Gently massage the scalp in circular motions to stimulate blood circulation and ensure even absorption.

4. **Leave-In:** Leave the treatment on for about 20-30 minutes. You can cover your hair with a shower cap for better penetration.

5. **Rinse:** Rinse your hair thoroughly with lukewarm water. You may use a mild sulfate-free shampoo if needed.

6. **Condition (Optional):** Depending on your hair type, you can follow up with a light conditioner, but avoid applying it to the scalp.

7. **Frequency:** Use this treatment once a week or as needed to help regulate oil production and maintain a refreshed scalp.

Balancing Castor Oil and Nettle Essential Oil Scalp Treatment for Oily Hair

Ingredients:

1. **Castor Oil (2 tablespoons):** Castor oil helps control excess oil production on the scalp.

2. **Jojoba Oil (1 tablespoon):** Jojoba oil helps balance oiliness without making the hair greasy.

3. **Nettle Essential Oil (7 drops):** Nettle oil is known for its astringent properties, which can help regulate oil production on the scalp.

4. **Lemon Juice (1 tablespoon):** Lemon juice cuts through excess oil and adds a refreshing scent.

5. **Aloe Vera Gel (1 tablespoon):** Aloe vera soothes the scalp, provides hydration, and helps maintain a healthy scalp balance.

Instructions:

1. **Mixing the Ingredients:** In a bowl, combine castor oil, jojoba oil, nettle essential oil, lemon juice, and aloe vera gel. Stir well to ensure all ingredients are thoroughly mixed.

2. **Application:** Section your hair and apply the mixture to

your scalp and roots, focusing on areas prone to oiliness. Use a brush or your fingertips to evenly distribute the treatment.

3. **Massage:** Gently massage the scalp in circular motions to stimulate blood circulation and ensure even absorption.

4. **Leave-In:** Leave the treatment on for about 20-30 minutes. You can cover your hair with a shower cap for better penetration.

5. **Rinse:** Rinse your hair thoroughly with lukewarm water. You may use a mild sulfate-free shampoo if needed.

6. **Condition (Optional):** Depending on your hair type, you can follow up with a light conditioner, but avoid applying it to the scalp.

7. **Frequency:** Use this treatment once a week or as needed to help regulate oil production and maintain a balanced scalp.

Purifying Castor Oil and Cedarwood Essential Oil Scalp Treatment for Oily Hair

Ingredients:

1. **Castor Oil (2 tablespoons):** Castor oil helps control excess oil production on the scalp.

2. **Argan Oil (1 tablespoon):** Argan oil is lightweight and helps balance oiliness without making the hair greasy.

3. **Cedarwood Essential Oil (8 drops):** Cedarwood oil has astringent properties that can help regulate oil production on the scalp.

4. **Lemon Juice (1 tablespoon):** Lemon juice cuts through excess oil and adds a refreshing scent.

5. **Aloe Vera Gel (1 tablespoon):** Aloe vera soothes the scalp, provides hydration, and helps maintain a healthy balance.

Instructions:

1. **Mixing the Ingredients:** In a bowl, combine castor oil, argan oil, cedarwood essential oil, lemon juice, and aloe vera gel. Stir well to ensure all ingredients are thoroughly mixed.

2. **Application:** Section your hair and apply the mixture to your scalp and roots, focusing on areas prone to oiliness. Use

a brush or your fingertips to evenly distribute the treatment.

3. **Massage:** Gently massage the scalp in circular motions to stimulate blood circulation and ensure even absorption.

4. **Leave-In:** Leave the treatment on for about 20-30 minutes. You can cover your hair with a shower cap for better penetration.

5. **Rinse:** Rinse your hair thoroughly with lukewarm water. You may use a mild sulfate-free shampoo if needed.

6. **Condition (Optional):** Depending on your hair type, you can follow up with a light conditioner, but avoid applying it to the scalp.

7. **Frequency:** Use this treatment once a week or as needed to help regulate oil production and maintain a balanced scalp.

Soothing Castor Oil and Jasmine Essential Oil Scalp Treatment for Oily Hair

Ingredients:

1. **Castor Oil (2 tablespoons):** Castor oil helps control excess oil production on the scalp.

2. **Sweet Almond Oil (1 tablespoon):** Sweet almond oil is lightweight and nourishing, balancing oiliness without making the hair greasy.

3. **Jasmine Essential Oil (6 drops):** Jasmine oil has soothing properties and adds a delightful floral fragrance.

4. **Lemon Juice (1 tablespoon):** Lemon juice cuts through excess oil and adds a refreshing scent.

5. **Aloe Vera Gel (1 tablespoon):** Aloe vera soothes the scalp, provides hydration, and helps maintain a healthy balance.

Instructions:

1. **Mixing the Ingredients:** In a bowl, combine castor oil, sweet almond oil, jasmine essential oil, lemon juice, and aloe vera gel. Stir well to ensure all ingredients are thoroughly mixed.

2. **Application:** Section your hair and apply the mixture to

your scalp and roots, focusing on areas prone to oiliness. Use a brush or your fingertips to evenly distribute the treatment.

3. **Massage:** Gently massage the scalp in circular motions to stimulate blood circulation and ensure even absorption.

4. **Leave-In:** Leave the treatment on for about 20-30 minutes. You can cover your hair with a shower cap for better penetration.

5. **Rinse:** Rinse your hair thoroughly with lukewarm water. You may use a mild sulfate-free shampoo if needed.

6. **Condition (Optional):** Depending on your hair type, you can follow up with a light conditioner, but avoid applying it to the scalp.

7. **Frequency:** Use this treatment once a week or as needed to help soothe the scalp, regulate oil production, and maintain a balanced environment.

Clarifying Castor Oil and Thyme Essential Oil Scalp Treatment for Oily Hair

Ingredients:

1. **Castor Oil (2 tablespoons):** Castor oil helps control excess oil production on the scalp.

2. **Grapeseed Oil (1 tablespoon):** Grapeseed oil is lightweight and helps balance oiliness without making the hair greasy.

3. **Thyme Essential Oil (7 drops):** Thyme oil has natural astringent properties that can assist in regulating oil production on the scalp.

4. **Lemon Juice (1 tablespoon):** Lemon juice cuts through excess oil and adds a refreshing scent.

5. **Aloe Vera Gel (1 tablespoon):** Aloe vera soothes the scalp, provides hydration, and helps maintain a healthy balance.

Instructions:

1. **Mixing the Ingredients:** In a bowl, combine castor oil, grapeseed oil, thyme essential oil, lemon juice, and aloe vera gel. Stir well to ensure all ingredients are thoroughly mixed.

2. **Application:** Section your hair and apply the mixture to your scalp and roots, focusing on areas prone to oiliness. Use

a brush or your fingertips to evenly distribute the treatment.

3. **Massage:** Gently massage the scalp in circular motions to stimulate blood circulation and ensure even absorption.

4. **Leave-In:** Leave the treatment on for about 20-30 minutes. You can cover your hair with a shower cap for better penetration.

5. **Rinse:** Rinse your hair thoroughly with lukewarm water. You may use a mild sulfate-free shampoo if needed.

6. **Condition (Optional):** Depending on your hair type, you can follow up with a light conditioner, but avoid applying it to the scalp.

7. **Frequency:** Use this treatment once a week or as needed to help clarify the scalp, control oiliness, and maintain a healthy balance.

CHAPTER THIRTEEN

Recipes for Dry Hair

Nourishing Castor Oil and Wheat Germ Oil Hair Mask for Dry Hair

Ingredients:

1. **Castor Oil (2 tablespoons):** Castor oil provides deep moisturization and helps nourish dry hair.

2. **Wheat Germ Oil (1 tablespoon):** Wheat germ oil is rich in vitamins and fatty acids, promoting hydration and overall hair health.

3. **Coconut Milk (2 tablespoons):** Coconut milk adds extra nourishment and helps condition dry hair.

4. **Honey (1 tablespoon):** Honey is a natural humectant, attracting and retaining moisture in the hair.

5. **Vanilla Extract (1/2 teaspoon):** Vanilla extract adds a pleasant fragrance to the mask.

Instructions:

1. **Mixing the Ingredients:** In a bowl, combine castor oil, wheat germ oil, coconut milk, honey, and vanilla extract. Mix well to create a smooth and uniform consistency.

2. **Application:** Dampen your hair slightly. Section your hair and apply the mixture from roots to ends, ensuring even coverage.

3. **Massage:** Gently massage the mask into your hair and scalp to enhance absorption and stimulate blood circulation.

4. **Wrap Hair:** Once applied, gather your hair and secure it in a bun. Cover your hair with a shower cap or a warm towel to create a heat-locking effect.

5. **Wait:** Leave the mask on for at least 30 minutes to allow the oils and nutrients to deeply penetrate the hair shaft.

6. **Rinse:** Rinse your hair thoroughly with lukewarm water. You can use a mild sulfate-free shampoo if needed.

7. **Condition (Optional):** Follow up with a conditioner if desired, focusing on the lengths and ends of your hair.

8. **Final Rinse:** For added shine, finish with a final rinse of cool water to seal the hair cuticles.

9. **Frequency:** Use this nourishing hair mask once a week or as needed to revive and hydrate dry hair.

Hydrating Castor Oil and Red Juniper Oil Hair Treatment for Dry Hair

Ingredients:

1. **Castor Oil (2 tablespoons):** Castor oil deeply moisturizes and nourishes dry hair.

2. **Argan Oil (1 tablespoon):** Argan oil is rich in nutrients and adds shine while moisturizing the hair.

3. **Red Juniper Essential Oil (6 drops):** Red juniper oil has soothing properties and adds a pleasant fragrance to the treatment.

4. **Avocado (1/2 mashed):** Avocado is rich in natural oils and vitamins, providing extra nourishment.

5. **Honey (1 tablespoon):** Honey is a humectant that attracts and retains moisture in the hair.

Instructions:

1. **Mixing the Ingredients:** In a bowl, combine castor oil, argan oil, red juniper essential oil, mashed avocado, and honey. Mix thoroughly to create a smooth, consistent blend.

2. **Application:** Dampen your hair slightly. Section your hair and apply the mixture from roots to ends, ensuring even

coverage.

3. **Massage:** Gently massage the treatment into your hair and scalp to enhance absorption and stimulate blood circulation.

4. **Wrap Hair:** Once applied, gather your hair and secure it in a bun. Cover your hair with a shower cap or a warm towel to create a heat-locking effect.

5. **Wait:** Leave the treatment on for at least 30-45 minutes to allow the oils and nutrients to deeply penetrate the hair shaft.

6. **Rinse:** Rinse your hair thoroughly with lukewarm water. You can use a mild sulfate-free shampoo if needed.

7. **Condition (Optional):** Follow up with a conditioner if desired, focusing on the lengths and ends of your hair.

8. **Final Rinse:** For added shine, finish with a final rinse of cool water to seal the hair cuticles.

9. **Frequency:** Use this hydrating hair treatment once a week or as needed to rejuvenate and moisturize dry hair.

Revitalizing Castor Oil and Bergamot Oil Hair Mask for Dry Hair

Ingredients:

1. **Castor Oil (2 tablespoons):** Castor oil deeply moisturizes and nourishes dry hair.

2. **Sweet Almond Oil (1 tablespoon):** Sweet almond oil adds additional hydration and promotes overall hair health.

3. **Bergamot Essential Oil (8 drops):** Bergamot oil has a refreshing and uplifting scent, promoting a revitalizing experience.

4. **Banana (1 ripe, mashed):** Banana is rich in natural oils and vitamins, providing extra nourishment.

5. **Honey (1 tablespoon):** Honey is a humectant that attracts and retains moisture in the hair.

Instructions:

1. **Mixing the Ingredients:** In a bowl, combine castor oil, sweet almond oil, bergamot essential oil, mashed banana, and honey. Mix thoroughly to create a smooth, consistent blend.

2. **Application:** Dampen your hair slightly. Section your hair

and apply the mixture from roots to ends, ensuring even coverage.

3. **Massage:** Gently massage the mask into your hair and scalp to enhance absorption and stimulate blood circulation.

4. **Wrap Hair:** Once applied, gather your hair and secure it in a bun. Cover your hair with a shower cap or a warm towel to create a heat-locking effect.

5. **Wait:** Leave the mask on for at least 30-45 minutes to allow the oils and nutrients to deeply penetrate the hair shaft.

6. **Rinse:** Rinse your hair thoroughly with lukewarm water. You can use a mild sulfate-free shampoo if needed.

7. **Condition (Optional):** Follow up with a conditioner if desired, focusing on the lengths and ends of your hair.

8. **Final Rinse:** For added shine, finish with a final rinse of cool water to seal the hair cuticles.

9. **Frequency:** Use this revitalizing hair mask once a week or as needed to rejuvenate and moisturize dry hair.

Egg Yolk and Castor Oil Hydrating Hair Mask for Dry Hair

Ingredients:

1. **Castor Oil (2 tablespoons):** Castor oil deeply moisturizes and nourishes dry hair.

2. **Coconut Oil (1 tablespoon):** Coconut oil adds extra hydration and promotes overall hair health.

3. **Egg Yolk (1):** Egg yolks are rich in proteins and fatty acids, providing essential nutrients for dry hair.

4. **Honey (1 tablespoon):** Honey is a humectant that attracts and retains moisture in the hair.

Instructions:

1. **Mixing the Ingredients:** In a bowl, whisk together castor oil, coconut oil, egg yolk, and honey until you achieve a smooth and uniform mixture.

2. **Application:** Dampen your hair slightly. Section your hair and apply the mixture from roots to ends, ensuring even coverage.

3. **Massage:** Gently massage the mask into your hair and scalp to enhance absorption and stimulate blood circulation.

4. **Wrap Hair:** Once applied, gather your hair and secure it in a bun. Cover your hair with a shower cap or a warm towel to create a heat-locking effect.

5. **Wait:** Leave the mask on for at least 30-45 minutes to allow the oils and nutrients to deeply penetrate the hair shaft.

6. **Rinse:** Rinse your hair thoroughly with lukewarm water. You can use a mild sulfate-free shampoo if needed.

7. **Condition (Optional):** Follow up with a conditioner if desired, focusing on the lengths and ends of your hair.

8. **Final Rinse:** For added shine, finish with a final rinse of cool water to seal the hair cuticles.

9. **Frequency:** Use this hydrating hair mask once a week or as needed to revive and moisturize dry hair.

Soothing Castor Oil and Sandalwood Oil Hair Treatment for Dry Hair

Ingredients:

1. **Castor Oil (2 tablespoons):** Castor oil deeply moisturizes and nourishes dry hair.

2. **Jojoba Oil (1 tablespoon):** Jojoba oil helps balance moisture and adds a lightweight shine to the hair.

3. **Sandalwood Essential Oil (6 drops):** Sandalwood oil has soothing properties and adds a delightful fragrance to the treatment.

4. **Avocado (1/2 mashed):** Avocado is rich in natural oils and vitamins, providing extra nourishment.

5. **Honey (1 tablespoon):** Honey is a humectant that attracts and retains moisture in the hair.

Instructions:

1. **Mixing the Ingredients:** In a bowl, combine castor oil, jojoba oil, sandalwood essential oil, mashed avocado, and honey. Mix thoroughly to create a smooth, consistent blend.

2. **Application:** Dampen your hair slightly. Section your hair and apply the mixture from roots to ends, ensuring even

coverage.

3. **Massage:** Gently massage the treatment into your hair and scalp to enhance absorption and stimulate blood circulation.

4. **Wrap Hair:** Once applied, gather your hair and secure it in a bun. Cover your hair with a shower cap or a warm towel to create a heat-locking effect.

5. **Wait:** Leave the treatment on for at least 30-45 minutes to allow the oils and nutrients to deeply penetrate the hair shaft.

6. **Rinse:** Rinse your hair thoroughly with lukewarm water. You can use a mild sulfate-free shampoo if needed.

7. **Condition (Optional):** Follow up with a conditioner if desired, focusing on the lengths and ends of your hair.

8. **Final Rinse:** For added shine, finish with a final rinse of cool water to seal the hair cuticles.

9. **Frequency:** Use this soothing hair treatment once a week or as needed to nourish and revive dry hair.

Nourishing Castor Oil and Bay Leaf Oil Hair Mask for Dry Hair

Ingredients:

1. **Castor Oil (2 tablespoons):** Castor oil deeply moisturizes and nourishes dry hair.

2. **Olive Oil (1 tablespoon):** Olive oil adds extra hydration and imparts a natural shine to the hair.

3. **Bay Leaf Essential Oil (7 drops):** Bay leaf oil has soothing properties and adds a fresh, herbal aroma to the treatment.

4. **Yogurt (2 tablespoons):** Yogurt is rich in proteins and helps in revitalizing and conditioning dry hair.

5. **Honey (1 tablespoon):** Honey is a humectant that attracts and retains moisture in the hair.

Instructions:

1. **Mixing the Ingredients:** In a bowl, combine castor oil, olive oil, bay leaf essential oil, yogurt, and honey. Mix thoroughly to create a smooth and consistent blend.

2. **Application:** Dampen your hair slightly. Section your hair and apply the mixture from roots to ends, ensuring even coverage.

3. **Massage:** Gently massage the mask into your hair and scalp to enhance absorption and stimulate blood circulation.

4. **Wrap Hair:** Once applied, gather your hair and secure it in a bun. Cover your hair with a shower cap or a warm towel to create a heat-locking effect.

5. **Wait:** Leave the mask on for at least 30-45 minutes to allow the oils and nutrients to deeply penetrate the hair shaft.

6. **Rinse:** Rinse your hair thoroughly with lukewarm water. You can use a mild sulfate-free shampoo if needed.

7. **Condition (Optional):** Follow up with a conditioner if desired, focusing on the lengths and ends of your hair.

8. **Final Rinse:** For added shine, finish with a final rinse of cool water to seal the hair cuticles.

9. **Frequency:** Use this nourishing hair mask once a week or as needed to revitalize and moisturize dry hair.

Moisturizing Castor Oil and Wintergreen Oil Hair Treatment for Dry Hair

Ingredients:

1. **Castor Oil (2 tablespoons):** Castor oil deeply moisturizes and nourishes dry hair.

2. **Coconut Oil (1 tablespoon):** Coconut oil adds extra hydration and promotes overall hair health.

3. **Wintergreen Essential Oil (5 drops):** Wintergreen oil has soothing properties and adds a refreshing scent to the treatment.

4. **Shea Butter (1 tablespoon, melted):** Shea butter is rich in vitamins and provides intense moisturization for dry hair.

5. **Aloe Vera Gel (1 tablespoon):** Aloe vera soothes the scalp, adds moisture, and helps maintain a healthy balance.

Instructions:

1. **Mixing the Ingredients:** In a bowl, combine castor oil, melted shea butter, coconut oil, wintergreen essential oil, and aloe vera gel. Mix thoroughly until you achieve a smooth, consistent blend.

2. **Application:** Dampen your hair slightly. Section your hair and apply the mixture from roots to ends, ensuring even coverage.

3. **Massage:** Gently massage the treatment into your hair and scalp to enhance absorption and stimulate blood circulation.

4. **Wrap Hair:** Once applied, gather your hair and secure it in a bun. Cover your hair with a shower cap or a warm towel to create a heat-locking effect.

5. **Wait:** Leave the treatment on for at least 30-45 minutes to allow the oils and nutrients to deeply penetrate the hair shaft.

6. **Rinse:** Rinse your hair thoroughly with lukewarm water. You can use a mild sulfate-free shampoo if needed.

7. **Condition (Optional):** Follow up with a conditioner if desired, focusing on the lengths and ends of your hair.

8. **Final Rinse:** For added shine, finish with a final rinse of cool water to seal the hair cuticles.

9. **Frequency:** Use this moisturizing hair treatment once a week or as needed to provide deep hydration for dry hair.

Revitalizing Castor Oil and Rosa Damascena Oil Hair Elixir for Dry Hair

Ingredients:

1. **Castor Oil (2 tablespoons):** Castor oil deeply moisturizes and nourishes dry hair.

2. **Argan Oil (1 tablespoon):** Argan oil adds extra hydration and promotes overall hair health.

3. **Rosa Damascena (Rose) Essential Oil (6 drops):** Rose oil has revitalizing properties and adds a luxurious floral aroma to the treatment.

4. **Avocado (1/2 mashed):** Avocado is rich in natural oils and vitamins, providing extra nourishment.

5. **Honey (1 tablespoon):** Honey is a humectant that attracts and retains moisture in the hair.

Instructions:

1. **Mixing the Ingredients:** In a bowl, combine castor oil, argan oil, rose essential oil, mashed avocado, and honey. Mix thoroughly until you achieve a smooth and consistent blend.

2. **Application:** Dampen your hair slightly. Section your hair and apply the mixture from roots to ends, ensuring even

coverage.

3. **Massage:** Gently massage the elixir into your hair and scalp to enhance absorption and stimulate blood circulation.

4. **Wrap Hair:** Once applied, gather your hair and secure it in a bun. Cover your hair with a shower cap or a warm towel to create a heat-locking effect.

5. **Wait:** Leave the elixir on for at least 30-45 minutes to allow the oils and nutrients to deeply penetrate the hair shaft.

6. **Rinse:** Rinse your hair thoroughly with lukewarm water. You can use a mild sulfate-free shampoo if needed.

7. **Condition (Optional):** Follow up with a conditioner if desired, focusing on the lengths and ends of your hair.

8. **Final Rinse:** For added shine, finish with a final rinse of cool water to seal the hair cuticles.

9. **Frequency:** Use this revitalizing hair elixir once a week or as needed to rejuvenate and moisturize dry hair.

Hydrating Castor Oil and Broccoli Seed Oil Hair Mask for Dry Hair

Ingredients:

1. **Castor Oil (2 tablespoons):** Castor oil deeply moisturizes and nourishes dry hair.

2. **Broccoli Seed Oil (1 tablespoon):** Broccoli seed oil is rich in fatty acids and vitamins, promoting hydration and shine.

3. **Coconut Milk (2 tablespoons):** Coconut milk adds extra nourishment and helps condition dry hair.

4. **Honey (1 tablespoon):** Honey is a humectant that attracts and retains moisture in the hair.

5. **Lavender Essential Oil (5 drops):** Lavender oil has calming properties and adds a pleasant fragrance to the mask.

Instructions:

1. **Mixing the Ingredients:** In a bowl, combine castor oil, broccoli seed oil, coconut milk, honey, and lavender essential oil. Mix thoroughly until you achieve a smooth and consistent blend.

2. **Application:** Dampen your hair slightly. Section your hair and apply the mixture from roots to ends, ensuring even

coverage.

3. **Massage:** Gently massage the mask into your hair and scalp to enhance absorption and stimulate blood circulation.

4. **Wrap Hair:** Once applied, gather your hair and secure it in a bun. Cover your hair with a shower cap or a warm towel to create a heat-locking effect.

5. **Wait:** Leave the mask on for at least 30-45 minutes to allow the oils and nutrients to deeply penetrate the hair shaft.

6. **Rinse:** Rinse your hair thoroughly with lukewarm water. You can use a mild sulfate-free shampoo if needed.

7. **Condition (Optional):** Follow up with a conditioner if desired, focusing on the lengths and ends of your hair.

8. **Final Rinse:** For added shine, finish with a final rinse of cool water to seal the hair cuticles.

9. **Frequency:** Use this hydrating hair mask once a week or as needed to provide deep nourishment for dry hair.

Revitalizing Castor Oil and Poppy Seed Oil Hair Treatment for Dry Hair

Ingredients:

1. **Castor Oil (2 tablespoons):** Castor oil deeply moisturizes and nourishes dry hair.

2. **Poppy Seed Oil (1 tablespoon):** Poppy seed oil is rich in essential fatty acids and adds shine while promoting hydration.

3. **Yogurt (2 tablespoons):** Yogurt provides proteins and helps revitalize and condition dry hair.

4. **Banana (1 ripe, mashed):** Banana is rich in natural oils and vitamins, providing extra nourishment.

5. **Geranium Essential Oil (5 drops):** Geranium oil has a floral fragrance and adds a luxurious touch to the treatment.

Instructions:

1. **Mixing the Ingredients:** In a bowl, combine castor oil, poppy seed oil, yogurt, mashed banana, and geranium essential oil. Mix thoroughly until you achieve a smooth and consistent blend.

2. **Application:** Dampen your hair slightly. Section your hair

and apply the mixture from roots to ends, ensuring even coverage.

3. **Massage:** Gently massage the treatment into your hair and scalp to enhance absorption and stimulate blood circulation.

4. **Wrap Hair:** Once applied, gather your hair and secure it in a bun. Cover your hair with a shower cap or a warm towel to create a heat-locking effect.

5. **Wait:** Leave the treatment on for at least 30-45 minutes to allow the oils and nutrients to deeply penetrate the hair shaft.

6. **Rinse:** Rinse your hair thoroughly with lukewarm water. You can use a mild sulfate-free shampoo if needed.

7. **Condition (Optional):** Follow up with a conditioner if desired, focusing on the lengths and ends of your hair.

8. **Final Rinse:** For added shine, finish with a final rinse of cool water to seal the hair cuticles.

9. **Frequency:** Use this revitalizing hair treatment once a week or as needed to rejuvenate and moisturize dry hair.

CHAPTER FOURTEEN

Recipes for Normal Hair

Balancing Castor Oil and Coconut Milk Hair Mask for Normal Hair

Ingredients:

1. **Castor Oil (2 tablespoons):** Castor oil promotes hair growth and provides essential nutrients.

2. **Coconut Milk (1/4 cup):** Coconut milk is rich in proteins and adds moisture, leaving hair soft and manageable.

3. **Aloe Vera Gel (2 tablespoons):** Aloe vera soothes the scalp,

maintains a healthy pH balance, and adds shine.

4. **Jojoba Oil (1 tablespoon):** Jojoba oil balances natural sebum production and nourishes the hair.

5. **Lemon Essential Oil (6 drops):** Lemon oil has a refreshing scent and helps maintain a clean and healthy scalp.

Instructions:

1. **Mixing the Ingredients:** In a bowl, combine castor oil, coconut milk, aloe vera gel, jojoba oil, and lemon essential oil. Mix well until all ingredients are thoroughly blended.

2. **Application:** Dampen your hair slightly. Section your hair and apply the mixture from roots to ends, ensuring even coverage.

3. **Massage:** Gently massage the mask into your hair and scalp to enhance absorption and stimulate blood circulation.

4. **Wrap Hair:** Once applied, gather your hair and secure it in a bun. Cover your hair with a shower cap or a warm towel to create a heat-locking effect.

5. **Wait:** Leave the mask on for 20-30 minutes to allow the nutrients to penetrate the hair shaft.

6. **Rinse:** Rinse your hair thoroughly with lukewarm water. You can use a mild sulfate-free shampoo if needed.

7. **Condition (Optional):** If desired, follow up with a condi-

tioner, focusing on the lengths and ends of your hair.

8. **Final Rinse:** For added shine, finish with a final rinse of cool water to seal the hair cuticles.

9. **Frequency:** Use this balancing hair mask once a week or as needed to maintain healthy and nourished normal hair.

Nourishing Castor Oil and Mimosa Absolute Hair Elixir for Normal Hair

Ingredients:

1. **Castor Oil (2 tablespoons):** Castor oil promotes hair growth and provides essential nutrients.

2. **Argan Oil (1 tablespoon):** Argan oil adds extra nourishment and imparts a natural shine to the hair.

3. **Mimosa Absolute Essential Oil (5 drops):** Mimosa absolute has a sweet, floral fragrance and adds a luxurious touch to the elixir.

4. **Avocado (1/2 mashed):** Avocado is rich in natural oils and vitamins, providing extra nourishment.

5. **Honey (1 tablespoon):** Honey is a humectant that attracts and retains moisture in the hair.

Instructions:

1. **Mixing the Ingredients:** In a bowl, combine castor oil, argan oil, mimosa absolute essential oil, mashed avocado, and honey. Mix thoroughly until you achieve a smooth and consistent blend.

2. **Application:** Dampen your hair slightly. Section your hair

and apply the elixir from roots to ends, ensuring even coverage.

3. **Massage:** Gently massage the elixir into your hair and scalp to enhance absorption and stimulate blood circulation.

4. **Wrap Hair:** Once applied, gather your hair and secure it in a bun. Cover your hair with a shower cap or a warm towel to create a heat-locking effect.

5. **Wait:** Leave the elixir on for at least 30-45 minutes to allow the oils and nutrients to deeply penetrate the hair shaft.

6. **Rinse:** Rinse your hair thoroughly with lukewarm water. You can use a mild sulfate-free shampoo if needed.

7. **Condition (Optional):** Follow up with a conditioner if desired, focusing on the lengths and ends of your hair.

8. **Final Rinse:** For added shine, finish with a final rinse of cool water to seal the hair cuticles.

9. **Frequency:** Use this nourishing hair elixir once a week or as needed to maintain healthy and nourished normal hair.

Balancing Castor Oil and Orange Blossom Absolute Hair Elixir for Normal Hair

Ingredients:

1. **Castor Oil (2 tablespoons):** Castor oil promotes hair growth and provides essential nutrients.

2. **Jojoba Oil (1 tablespoon):** Jojoba oil helps balance moisture and adds a lightweight shine to the hair.

3. **Orange Blossom (Neroli) Absolute (5 drops):** Orange blossom absolute has a sweet, floral fragrance and adds a luxurious aroma to the elixir.

4. **Coconut Milk (2 tablespoons):** Coconut milk adds extra nourishment and helps condition normal hair.

5. **Aloe Vera Gel (1 tablespoon):** Aloe vera soothes the scalp, maintains a healthy pH balance, and adds shine.

Instructions:

1. **Mixing the Ingredients:** In a bowl, combine castor oil, jojoba oil, orange blossom absolute, coconut milk, and aloe vera gel. Mix thoroughly until you achieve a smooth and consistent blend.

2. **Application:** Dampen your hair slightly. Section your hair and apply the elixir from roots to ends, ensuring even coverage.

3. **Massage:** Gently massage the elixir into your hair and scalp to enhance absorption and stimulate blood circulation.

4. **Wrap Hair:** Once applied, gather your hair and secure it in a bun. Cover your hair with a shower cap or a warm towel to create a heat-locking effect.

5. **Wait:** Leave the elixir on for at least 30-45 minutes to allow the oils and nutrients to deeply penetrate the hair shaft.

6. **Rinse:** Rinse your hair thoroughly with lukewarm water. You can use a mild sulfate-free shampoo if needed.

7. **Condition (Optional):** Follow up with a conditioner if desired, focusing on the lengths and ends of your hair.

8. **Final Rinse:** For added shine, finish with a final rinse of cool water to seal the hair cuticles.

9. **Frequency:** Use this balancing hair elixir once a week or as needed to maintain healthy and nourished normal hair.

Revitalizing Castor Oil and Fresh Papaya Juice Hair Mask for Normal Hair

Ingredients:

1. **Castor Oil (2 tablespoons):** Castor oil promotes hair growth and provides essential nutrients.

2. **Fresh Papaya Juice (1/4 cup):** Papaya is rich in vitamins and enzymes that nourish and condition the hair.

3. **Honey (1 tablespoon):** Honey is a humectant that attracts and retains moisture in the hair.

4. **Coconut Oil (1 tablespoon):** Coconut oil adds extra hydration and promotes overall hair health.

5. **Lemon Juice (1 tablespoon):** Lemon juice helps balance the scalp's pH and adds a natural shine.

Instructions:

1. **Mixing the Ingredients:** In a bowl, combine castor oil, fresh papaya juice, honey, coconut oil, and lemon juice. Mix thoroughly until you achieve a smooth and consistent blend.

2. **Application:** Dampen your hair slightly. Section your hair and apply the mask from roots to ends, ensuring even coverage.

3. **Massage:** Gently massage the mask into your hair and scalp to enhance absorption and stimulate blood circulation.

4. **Wrap Hair:** Once applied, gather your hair and secure it in a bun. Cover your hair with a shower cap or a warm towel to create a heat-locking effect.

5. **Wait:** Leave the mask on for 30-45 minutes to allow the nutrients to deeply penetrate the hair shaft.

6. **Rinse:** Rinse your hair thoroughly with lukewarm water. You can use a mild sulfate-free shampoo if needed.

7. **Condition (Optional):** Follow up with a conditioner if desired, focusing on the lengths and ends of your hair.

8. **Final Rinse:** For added shine, finish with a final rinse of cool water to seal the hair cuticles.

9. **Frequency:** Use this revitalizing hair mask once a week or as needed to maintain healthy and nourished normal hair.

Balancing Castor Oil and Meadowsweet Hair Rinse for Normal Hair

Ingredients:

1. **Castor Oil (1 tablespoon):** Castor oil promotes hair growth and provides essential nutrients.

2. **Meadowsweet Infusion (1 cup):** Meadowsweet is known for its balancing properties and helps maintain a healthy scalp.

3. **Apple Cider Vinegar (2 tablespoons):** Apple cider vinegar helps balance the hair's pH and adds shine.

4. **Rosemary Essential Oil (5 drops):** Rosemary oil stimulates the scalp and promotes overall hair health.

Instructions:

1. **Prepare Meadowsweet Infusion:**

   - Boil 1 cup of water and pour it over 1-2 tablespoons of dried meadowsweet flowers.

   - Allow the mixture to steep for 15-20 minutes, then strain to obtain meadowsweet infusion.

2. **Mixing the Ingredients:**

- In a bowl, combine castor oil, meadowsweet infusion, apple cider vinegar, and rosemary essential oil. Mix well.

3. **Application:**

- After shampooing, pour the mixture over your hair, ensuring even distribution.

4. **Massage:**

- Gently massage the mixture into your scalp for a few minutes to stimulate blood circulation.

5. **Wait:**

- Leave the rinse on for 5-10 minutes to allow the properties to work on your hair and scalp.

6. **Rinse:**

- Rinse your hair thoroughly with lukewarm water.

7. **Final Rinse:**

- Optionally, you can do a final rinse with cool water to seal the hair cuticles.

8. **Frequency:**

- Use this meadowsweet hair rinse once a week or as needed to maintain a balanced and healthy scalp.

Nourishing Castor Oil and Angelica Root Oil Hair Elixir for Normal Hair

Ingredients:

1. **Castor Oil (2 tablespoons):** Castor oil promotes hair growth and provides essential nutrients.

2. **Angelica Root Essential Oil (5 drops):** Angelica root oil nourishes the hair and adds a herbal aroma to the elixir.

3. **Sweet Almond Oil (1 tablespoon):** Sweet almond oil adds extra nourishment and promotes overall hair health.

4. **Honey (1 tablespoon):** Honey is a humectant that attracts and retains moisture in the hair.

5. **Chamomile Tea (1/4 cup, cooled):** Chamomile tea soothes the scalp and adds a calming effect.

Instructions:

1. **Mixing the Ingredients:**

   - In a bowl, combine castor oil, angelica root essential oil, sweet almond oil, honey, and cooled chamomile tea. Mix thoroughly until you achieve a smooth and consistent blend.

2. **Application:**

- Dampen your hair slightly. Section your hair and apply the elixir from roots to ends, ensuring even coverage.

3. **Massage:**

- Gently massage the elixir into your hair and scalp to enhance absorption and stimulate blood circulation.

4. **Wrap Hair:**

- Once applied, gather your hair and secure it in a bun. Cover your hair with a shower cap or a warm towel to create a heat-locking effect.

5. **Wait:**

- Leave the elixir on for at least 30-45 minutes to allow the oils and nutrients to deeply penetrate the hair shaft.

6. **Rinse:**

- Rinse your hair thoroughly with lukewarm water. You can use a mild sulfate-free shampoo if needed.

7. **Condition (Optional):**

- Follow up with a conditioner if desired, focusing on the lengths and ends of your hair.

8. **Final Rinse:**

- For added shine, finish with a final rinse of cool water to seal the hair cuticles.

9. Frequency:

- Use this nourishing hair elixir once a week or as needed to maintain healthy and nourished normal hair.

Soothing Castor Oil and Licorice Root Oil Hair Elixir for Normal Hair

Ingredients:

1. **Castor Oil (2 tablespoons):** Castor oil promotes hair growth and provides essential nutrients.

2. **Licorice Root Essential Oil (5 drops):** Licorice root oil soothes the scalp and adds a subtle herbal fragrance to the elixir.

3. **Jojoba Oil (1 tablespoon):** Jojoba oil balances natural sebum production and nourishes the hair.

4. **Yogurt (2 tablespoons):** Yogurt provides proteins and helps condition normal hair.

5. **Peppermint Tea (1/4 cup, cooled):** Peppermint tea adds a refreshing sensation and promotes scalp health.

Instructions:

1. **Mixing the Ingredients:**

   - In a bowl, combine castor oil, licorice root essential oil, jojoba oil, yogurt, and cooled peppermint tea. Mix thoroughly until you achieve a smooth and consistent blend.

2. **Application:**

- Dampen your hair slightly. Section your hair and apply the elixir from roots to ends, ensuring even coverage.

3. **Massage:**

- Gently massage the elixir into your hair and scalp to enhance absorption and stimulate blood circulation.

4. **Wrap Hair:**

- Once applied, gather your hair and secure it in a bun. Cover your hair with a shower cap or a warm towel to create a heat-locking effect.

5. **Wait:**

- Leave the elixir on for at least 30-45 minutes to allow the oils and nutrients to deeply penetrate the hair shaft.

6. **Rinse:**

- Rinse your hair thoroughly with lukewarm water. You can use a mild sulfate-free shampoo if needed.

7. **Condition (Optional):**

- Follow up with a conditioner if desired, focusing on the lengths and ends of your hair.

8. **Final Rinse:**

- For added shine, finish with a final rinse of cool water to seal the hair cuticles.

9. **Frequency:**

- Use this soothing hair elixir once a week or as needed to maintain a healthy and balanced scalp.

Balancing Castor Oil and Palmarosa Oil Hair Elixir for Normal Hair

Ingredients:

1. **Castor Oil (2 tablespoons):** Castor oil promotes hair growth and provides essential nutrients.

2. **Palmarosa Essential Oil (5 drops):** Palmarosa oil balances oil production and adds a floral fragrance to the elixir.

3. **Argan Oil (1 tablespoon):** Argan oil adds extra nourishment and imparts a natural shine to the hair.

4. **Aloe Vera Gel (2 tablespoons):** Aloe vera soothes the scalp, maintains a healthy pH balance, and adds hydration.

5. **Green Tea (1/4 cup, cooled):** Green tea helps revitalize the hair and provides antioxidants.

Instructions:

1. **Mixing the Ingredients:**

   - In a bowl, combine castor oil, palmarosa essential oil, argan oil, aloe vera gel, and cooled green tea. Mix thoroughly until you achieve a smooth and consistent blend.

2. **Application:**

- Dampen your hair slightly. Section your hair and apply the elixir from roots to ends, ensuring even coverage.

3. **Massage:**

- Gently massage the elixir into your hair and scalp to enhance absorption and stimulate blood circulation.

4. **Wrap Hair:**

- Once applied, gather your hair and secure it in a bun. Cover your hair with a shower cap or a warm towel to create a heat-locking effect.

5. **Wait:**

- Leave the elixir on for at least 30-45 minutes to allow the oils and nutrients to deeply penetrate the hair shaft.

6. **Rinse:**

- Rinse your hair thoroughly with lukewarm water. You can use a mild sulfate-free shampoo if needed.

7. **Condition (Optional):**

- Follow up with a conditioner if desired, focusing on the lengths and ends of your hair.

8. **Final Rinse:**

- For added shine, finish with a final rinse of cool water to seal the hair cuticles.

9. **Frequency:**

- Use this balancing hair elixir once a week or as needed to maintain healthy and nourished normal hair.

Nourishing Castor Oil and Marshmallow Root Oil Hair Elixir for Normal Hair

Ingredients:

1. **Castor Oil (2 tablespoons):** Castor oil promotes hair growth and provides essential nutrients.

2. **Marshmallow Root Essential Oil (5 drops):** Marshmallow root oil nourishes the hair and adds a subtle herbal fragrance to the elixir.

3. **Sweet Almond Oil (1 tablespoon):** Sweet almond oil adds extra nourishment and promotes overall hair health.

4. **Honey (1 tablespoon):** Honey is a humectant that attracts and retains moisture in the hair.

5. **Chamomile Tea (1/4 cup, cooled):** Chamomile tea soothes the scalp and adds a calming effect.

Instructions:

1. **Mixing the Ingredients:**

   - In a bowl, combine castor oil, marshmallow root essential oil, sweet almond oil, honey, and cooled chamomile tea. Mix thoroughly until you achieve a smooth and consistent blend.

2. **Application:**

- Dampen your hair slightly. Section your hair and apply the elixir from roots to ends, ensuring even coverage.

3. **Massage:**

- Gently massage the elixir into your hair and scalp to enhance absorption and stimulate blood circulation.

4. **Wrap Hair:**

- Once applied, gather your hair and secure it in a bun. Cover your hair with a shower cap or a warm towel to create a heat-locking effect.

5. **Wait:**

- Leave the elixir on for at least 30-45 minutes to allow the oils and nutrients to deeply penetrate the hair shaft.

6. **Rinse:**

- Rinse your hair thoroughly with lukewarm water. You can use a mild sulfate-free shampoo if needed.

7. **Condition (Optional):**

- Follow up with a conditioner if desired, focusing on the lengths and ends of your hair.

8. **Final Rinse:**

- For added shine, finish with a final rinse of cool water to seal the hair cuticles.

9. **Frequency:**

- Use this nourishing hair elixir once a week or as needed to maintain healthy and nourished normal hair.

Vibrant Castor Oil and Fresh Strawberry Juice Hair Mask for Normal Hair

Ingredients:

1. **Castor Oil (2 tablespoons):** Castor oil promotes hair growth and provides essential nutrients.

2. **Fresh Strawberry Juice (1/4 cup):** Strawberries are rich in vitamins and antioxidants that nourish the hair.

3. **Coconut Milk (2 tablespoons):** Coconut milk adds extra nourishment and helps condition normal hair.

4. **Honey (1 tablespoon):** Honey is a humectant that attracts and retains moisture in the hair.

5. **Jojoba Oil (1 tablespoon):** Jojoba oil balances natural sebum production and nourishes the hair.

Instructions:

1. **Preparing Strawberry Juice:**

   - Blend fresh strawberries to extract juice. Strain to remove pulp, obtaining fresh strawberry juice.

2. **Mixing the Ingredients:**

   - In a bowl, combine castor oil, fresh strawberry juice,

coconut milk, honey, and jojoba oil. Mix thoroughly until you achieve a smooth and consistent blend.

3. **Application:**

- Dampen your hair slightly. Section your hair and apply the mask from roots to ends, ensuring even coverage.

4. **Massage:**

- Gently massage the mask into your hair and scalp to enhance absorption and stimulate blood circulation.

5. **Wrap Hair:**

- Once applied, gather your hair and secure it in a bun. Cover your hair with a shower cap or a warm towel to create a heat-locking effect.

6. **Wait:**

- Leave the mask on for 30-45 minutes to allow the nutrients to deeply penetrate the hair shaft.

7. **Rinse:**

- Rinse your hair thoroughly with lukewarm water. You can use a mild sulfate-free shampoo if needed.

8. **Condition (Optional):**

- Follow up with a conditioner if desired, focusing on the lengths and ends of your hair.

9. **Final Rinse:**

- For added shine, finish with a final rinse of cool water to seal the hair cuticles.

10. **Frequency:**

- Use this vibrant hair mask once a week or as needed to maintain healthy and nourished normal hair.

CHAPTER FIFTEEN

Remedies with Castor Oil

J ust as a skilled alchemist combines elements to create powerful elixirs, here you can find a curated set of remedies that harness the potent properties of castor oil. From eyelash serum to joint health, each recipe is a testament to the holistic approach of embracing nature's bounty for optimal health.

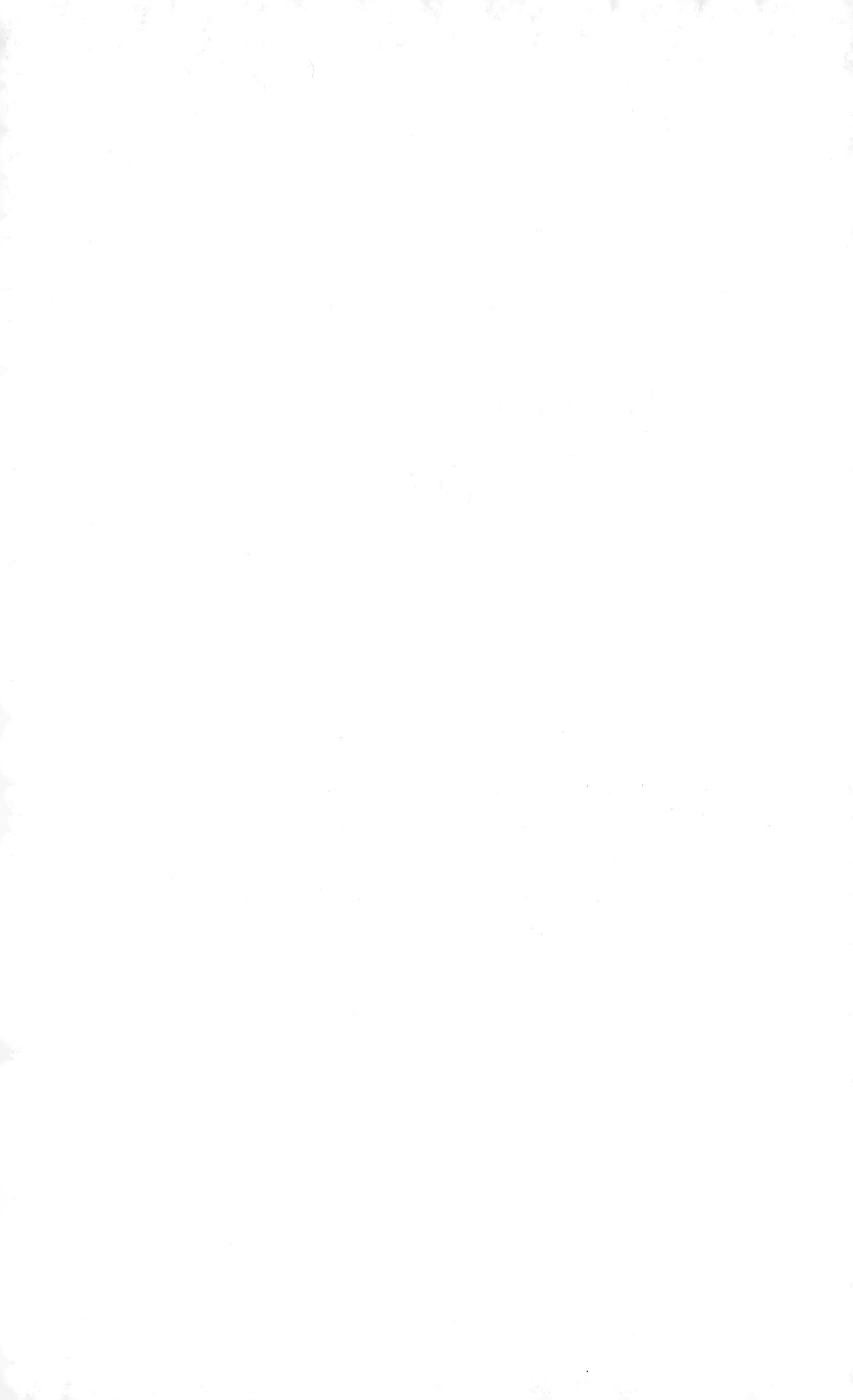

CHAPTER SIXTEEN

DIY Remedies

Natural Eyelash and Eyebrow Growth Serum with Castor Oil

Ingredients:

1. **Castor Oil (1 tablespoon):** Castor oil is known to promote hair growth and strengthen hair follicles.

2. **Sweet Almond Oil (1/2 tablespoon):** Sweet almond oil nourishes and conditions the lashes and eyebrows.

Instructions:

1. **Mixing the Ingredients:**

   - In a small, clean glass container, combine castor oil with sweet almond oil. Mix well using a clean utensil.

2. **Application:**

   - Using a clean mascara wand or a cotton swab, apply a small amount of the serum to your eyelashes and eyebrows.

3. **Massage:**

   - Gently massage the serum into the lashes and brows using your fingertips for a few minutes.

4. **Frequency:**

   - Apply the serum every night before bedtime for the best results. Consistency is key.

5. **Avoid Contact with Eyes:**

   - Be cautious not to let the serum come into direct contact with your eyes.

6. **Store in a Cool Place:**

   - Store the serum in a cool, dark place to preserve its effectiveness.

Note: Patch test the serum on a small area of your skin before applying it to your eyelashes and eyebrows to ensure you don't have any adverse reactions.

Invigorating Hair Growth Treatment with Castor Oil and Rosemary Oil

Ingredients:

1. **Castor Oil (2 tablespoons):** Castor oil is rich in nutrients and promotes hair growth.

2. **Jojoba Oil (1 tablespoon):** Jojoba oil nourishes the hair follicles and adds shine.

3. **Rosemary Essential Oil (10 drops):** Rosemary oil stimulates blood circulation to the scalp and encourages hair growth.

4. **Peppermint Essential Oil (5 drops):** Peppermint oil has a cooling effect and supports hair follicle health.

5. **Lavender Essential Oil (5 drops):** Lavender oil has calming properties and promotes a healthy scalp.

Instructions:

1. **Mixing the Ingredients:**

   - In a small, clean glass bottle, combine castor oil, jojoba oil, rosemary essential oil, peppermint essential oil, and lavender essential oil. Shake well to ensure thorough mixing.

2. **Application:**

- Part your hair and apply the mixture directly to the scalp using the dropper or your fingertips.

3. **Massage:**

- Gently massage the oil blend into your scalp using circular motions. Ensure even distribution.

4. **Application to Hair Length (Optional):**

- If desired, apply a small amount of the mixture to the lengths of your hair for extra nourishment.

5. **Wrap Hair (Optional):**

- For a deep treatment, wrap your hair in a warm towel or use a shower cap to create heat and enhance absorption.

6. **Wait:**

- Leave the treatment on for at least 30 minutes or, for a deeper treatment, leave it on overnight.

7. **Shampoo and Condition:**

- Wash your hair thoroughly with a mild sulfate-free shampoo and conditioner.

8. **Frequency:**

- Use this treatment 1-2 times a week for optimal results.

Soothing Joint Pain Relief Balm with Castor Oil

Ingredients:

1. **Castor Oil (2 tablespoons):** Castor oil has anti-inflammatory properties and penetrates deeply to soothe joint pain.

2. **Beeswax (1 tablespoon, grated or pellets):** Beeswax adds thickness and helps the balm solidify. It also forms a protective barrier on the skin.

3. **Peppermint Essential Oil (5 drops):** Peppermint oil provides a cooling sensation, which can help alleviate pain and discomfort.

4. **Eucalyptus Essential Oil (5 drops):** Eucalyptus oil is known for its analgesic and anti-inflammatory properties, making it beneficial for relieving joint pain.

Instructions:

1. **Prepare a Double Boiler:**

   - Fill a small saucepan with water and bring it to a simmer. Place a heat-safe bowl over the saucepan, creating a double boiler.

2. **Melt Beeswax:**

   - Add the grated or pelletized beeswax to the bowl and let

it melt. Stir occasionally to ensure even melting.

3. **Add Castor Oil:**

   ○ Once the beeswax is melted, add the castor oil to the bowl. Continue stirring until the two ingredients are well combined.

4. **Incorporate Essential Oils:**

   ○ Remove the bowl from heat and let the mixture cool slightly. Add the drops of peppermint and eucalyptus essential oils. Stir thoroughly to distribute the oils evenly.

5. **Pour into Containers:**

   ○ Pour the mixture into small, clean containers or tins. Allow it to cool and solidify completely.

6. **Application:**

   ○ Take a small amount of the balm and massage it onto the affected joints. The balm will melt slightly upon contact with the skin, making it easy to apply.

7. **Store in a Cool Place:**

   ○ Keep the joint pain relief balm in a cool place to prevent it from melting. A cool, dark cupboard or the refrigerator is ideal.

8. **Use as Needed:**

   ○ Apply the balm to sore joints whenever you experience

pain or inflammation. It can be used multiple times throughout the day as needed.

Note: While this balm may provide relief for mild joint pain, it's important to consult with a healthcare professional for persistent or severe joint issues. Additionally, perform a patch test before widespread application to ensure you don't have any adverse reactions to the essential oils.

Hydrating Lip Balm Recipe with Castor Oil

Ingredients:

1. **Castor Oil (1 tablespoon):** Castor oil is a thick, emollient oil that helps lock in moisture and provides a protective barrier for the lips.

2. **Coconut Oil (1 tablespoon):** Coconut oil is rich in fatty acids, offering deep hydration and promoting soft, supple lips.

3. **Beeswax (1 tablespoon, grated or pellets):** Beeswax provides structure to the lip balm, helping it solidify and stay in place. It also forms a protective layer on the lips.

4. **Honey (1 teaspoon):** Honey is a natural humectant, attracting and retaining moisture to keep the lips hydrated. It also adds a subtle sweetness.

Instructions:

1. **Prepare a Double Boiler:**

   - Set up a double boiler by filling a small saucepan with water and placing a heat-safe bowl on top. Bring the water to a simmer.

2. **Combine Ingredients:**

- In the bowl, combine castor oil, coconut oil, and grated or pelletized beeswax. Stir the mixture until the ingredients are well combined.

3. Melt and Blend:

- Allow the ingredients to melt completely, stirring occasionally. Once melted, add honey to the mixture and blend thoroughly.

4. Check Consistency:

- To check the consistency, place a small drop of the mixture on a cold spoon. If it solidifies quickly, it's ready.

5. Pour into Containers:

- Pour the liquid lip balm into small, clean containers or lip balm tubes. Work quickly before the mixture solidifies.

6. Cool and Solidify:

- Let the lip balm cool and solidify at room temperature or, for a faster setting, place it in the refrigerator for about 30 minutes.

7. Apply as Needed:

- Use your finger or a lip brush to apply the balm to your lips whenever they feel dry or chapped. The balm will melt slightly upon contact with the warmth of your lips.

8. Store in a Cool Place:

- ○ Keep the lip balm in a cool place to maintain its structure. If using tubes, avoid leaving them in direct sunlight or heat.

Scar Reduction Oil with Castor Oil

Ingredients:

1. **Castor Oil (2 tablespoons):** Castor oil's thick consistency and moisturizing properties make it beneficial for scar reduction.

2. **Vitamin E Oil (1 teaspoon):** Vitamin E is known for its skin-healing properties and helps improve the texture and appearance of scars.

Instructions:

1. **Combine Ingredients:**

   - In a small, clean bowl, mix together the castor oil and vitamin E oil. Stir well to ensure a homogenous blend.

2. **Cleanse the Skin:**

   - Before applying the scar reduction oil, cleanse the area around the scar with a gentle cleanser. Pat the skin dry.

3. **Apply the Mixture:**

   - Using a clean fingertip or cotton swab, apply a small amount of the oil mixture directly to the scar. Gently massage the oil into the skin using circular motions.

4. **Massage Technique:**

- Massage the scar for about 5-10 minutes. Massaging promotes blood circulation, which may aid in the absorption of the oils and help reduce scar tissue.

5. **Leave Overnight (Optional):**

- For a deeper treatment, you can leave the scar reduction oil on overnight. Cover the treated area with a clean bandage or gauze to prevent staining of clothing or bedding.

6. **Repeat Regularly:**

- For optimal results, apply the scar reduction oil regularly, preferably once or twice daily. Consistency is key when working on scar reduction.

7. **Sun Protection:**

- If the scar is exposed to the sun, ensure you use sunscreen with a high SPF to protect the healing skin from UV damage.

8. **Patience and Time:**

- Reduction of scars takes time, and individual results may vary. Be patient and continue the application until you notice an improvement in the appearance of the scar.

Nourishing Nail and Cuticle Treatment with Castor Oil

Ingredients:

1. **Castor Oil (1 tablespoon):** Castor oil is rich in nutrients and fatty acids that promote strong and healthy nails.

2. **Argan Oil (1 tablespoon):** Argan oil is a lightweight, nourishing oil that helps moisturize the nails and cuticles.

Instructions:

1. **Combine Oils:**

   - In a small bowl or a dropper bottle, mix together the castor oil and argan oil. Stir or shake well to ensure the oils are thoroughly combined.

2. **Cleanse Nails and Cuticles:**

   - Before applying the treatment, wash your hands and cleanse your nails and cuticles to remove any dirt or residue.

3. **Apply the Oil Mixture:**

   - Using a clean dropper or your fingertips, apply a small amount of the oil mixture to each nail and massage it into the cuticles.

4. **Massage Technique:**

- Gently massage the oil into the nails and cuticles in circular motions. Massaging helps improve blood circulation, promoting better nutrient absorption.

5. **Leave On:**

- Allow the oil mixture to remain on your nails and cuticles for at least 15-20 minutes. For a more intensive treatment, you can leave it on overnight by wearing cotton gloves.

6. **Repeat Regularly:**

- For optimal results, repeat the nail and cuticle treatment regularly. Aim to do this at least 2-3 times a week, or as needed, to keep your nails and cuticles well-nourished.

7. **Protect Your Nails:**

- Wear gloves when doing household chores or tasks that may expose your nails to harsh chemicals or excessive water to protect them from damage.

8. **Trim and Shape:**

- Maintain your nails by regularly trimming and shaping them. This, combined with the nourishing treatment, can contribute to healthier, stronger nails.

Note: If you have any nail or cuticle infections or concerns, consult with a dermatologist before starting a new nail care routine. Additionally, be consistent with your nail care practices for the best results over time.

DIY Natural Deodorant Balm with Castor Oil

Ingredients:

1. **Castor Oil (2 tablespoons):** Castor oil provides a smooth and moisturizing base for the deodorant balm.

2. **Baking Soda (1 tablespoon):** Baking soda helps neutralize odors and acts as a natural deodorizer.

3. **Cornstarch (1 tablespoon):** Cornstarch helps absorb moisture, keeping your underarms feeling dry.

4. **Essential Oil (a few drops):** Choose your favorite essential oil for a pleasant scent and additional antimicrobial properties. Lavender and tea tree oil are popular choices.

Instructions:

1. **Mix Dry Ingredients:**

   ○ In a clean bowl, combine baking soda and cornstarch. Stir well to ensure an even distribution of both ingredients.

2. **Add Castor Oil:**

   ○ Pour the castor oil into the dry ingredients. Mix thoroughly until you achieve a smooth, paste-like consistency.

3. **Add Essential Oil:**

- Add a few drops of your chosen essential oil (lavender, tea tree, etc.) to the mixture. Stir well to evenly distribute the scent.

4. **Adjust Consistency (Optional):**

- If the mixture is too thick, you can add a bit more castor oil. If it's too runny, add a small amount of baking soda or cornstarch until you reach the desired consistency.

5. **Transfer to Container:**

- Transfer the deodorant balm into a clean, airtight container. A small jar or an empty deodorant container works well.

6. **Cool and Solidify:**

- Allow the deodorant balm to cool and solidify at room temperature or in the refrigerator if you want to speed up the process.

7. **Application:**

- Using clean fingers, scoop a small amount of the balm and apply it to clean underarms. Massage gently until the balm is absorbed.

8. **Store in a Cool Place:**

- Keep the deodorant balm in a cool place to maintain its structure. If the weather is warm, you may store it in the refrigerator to prevent melting.

Note: As with any new product, perform a patch test to ensure you don't have any adverse reactions, especially if you have sensitive skin. This natural deodorant balm offers a gentle and effective alternative to commercial deodorants, keeping your underarms feeling fresh throughout the day.

Soothing Heel Balm with Castor Oil

Ingredients:

1. **Castor Oil (2 tablespoons):** Castor oil's moisturizing properties penetrate deeply, providing intense hydration for dry and cracked skin.

2. **Shea Butter (1 tablespoon):** Shea butter is rich in fatty acids and vitamins, contributing to the balm's nourishing and softening effects.

3. **Peppermint Essential Oil (5 drops):** Peppermint oil adds a refreshing and cooling sensation to the balm. It also has antibacterial properties that can benefit the feet.

Instructions:

1. **Melt Shea Butter:**

   - In a heat-safe bowl or double boiler, melt the shea butter until it becomes a liquid. Ensure it cools slightly before moving to the next step.

2. **Add Castor Oil:**

   - Once the shea butter is melted, add the castor oil to the bowl. Stir well to combine the two ingredients thoroughly.

3. Incorporate Peppermint Essential Oil:

- Allow the mixture to cool a bit more before adding the drops of peppermint essential oil. Stir to evenly distribute the refreshing aroma.

4. Cool and Solidify:

- Let the mixture cool until it begins to solidify but is still spreadable. This ensures a comfortable application.

5. Transfer to Container:

- Transfer the balm into a clean, airtight container. A jar with a tight lid works well for easy storage and application.

6. Application Before Bed:

- Before bedtime, wash and thoroughly dry your feet. Scoop out a small amount of the balm and massage it onto your heels and any other dry areas on your feet.

7. Cover with Socks:

- To enhance the absorption of the balm, cover your treated feet with clean socks before going to bed. This creates a gentle occlusive effect, allowing the balm to work its magic overnight.

8. Wake Up to Softer Feet:

- In the morning, remove the socks and enjoy the feeling of smoother, more hydrated feet. If needed, wash your feet to remove any excess balm.

Note: For individuals with sensitive skin, perform a patch test before using the balm on a larger area. Regular use of this softening heel balm can help maintain the health and appearance of your feet, particularly in dry or colder seasons.

Soothing Massage Oil for Sore Muscles with Castor Oil

Ingredients:

1. **Castor Oil (2 tablespoons):** Castor oil's anti-inflammatory properties can help reduce muscle soreness and promote relaxation.

2. **Warming Essential Oil (10 drops):** Choose a warming essential oil such as ginger or black pepper. These oils can enhance circulation and provide a comforting sensation when applied to sore muscles.

Instructions:

1. **Mix the Oils:**

   - In a small bowl or a dark-colored glass bottle, combine the castor oil with the chosen warming essential oil. Stir or shake well to ensure the oils are evenly blended.

2. **Test Sensitivity:**

   - Perform a patch test on a small area of skin to ensure you don't have any adverse reactions to the essential oil. Wait 24 hours before applying the blend more extensively.

3. **Warm the Oil (Optional):**

   - For an added soothing effect, you can warm the massage

oil slightly. Place the container in a bowl of warm water or run it under warm tap water for a few minutes. Do not microwave the oil, as it may degrade the properties of the essential oil.

4. **Apply to Sore Muscles:**

   ○ Take a small amount of the massage oil and apply it to the sore muscles. Gently massage the oil into the skin using circular motions and firm, but not too intense, pressure.

5. **Focus on Trouble Areas:**

   ○ Concentrate on the areas with muscle tension or soreness. Allow the oil to be absorbed as you massage, promoting relaxation and comfort.

6. **Post-Massage Relaxation:**

   ○ After massaging, take a moment to relax and allow the oils to continue working. You can cover the treated area with a warm towel for added comfort.

7. **Repeat as Needed:**

   ○ Use this soothing massage oil as needed to alleviate muscle soreness. It's ideal after a workout or a long day of physical activity.

8. **Storage:**

   ○ Store the massage oil in a cool, dark place to preserve the integrity of the oils. Ensure the container is tightly sealed.

Note: If you have any existing medical conditions or concerns, consult with a healthcare professional before using this massage oil. Adjust the essential oil concentration based on personal preference and skin sensitivity.

Gentle Makeup Remover with Castor Oil and Jojoba Oil

Ingredients:

1. **Castor Oil (2 tablespoons):** Castor oil's emollient properties help break down and dissolve makeup while moisturizing the skin.

2. **Jojoba Oil (1 tablespoon):** Jojoba oil is a lightweight and non-greasy oil that mimics the skin's natural oils, making it an excellent choice for cleansing.

Instructions:

1. **Mix the Oils:**

   - In a small, clean bottle or container, combine the castor oil with the jojoba oil. Gently shake or stir to ensure the oils are well-mixed.

2. **Test Sensitivity:**

   - Before using the makeup remover on your entire face, perform a patch test on a small area to check for any adverse reactions. Wait 24 hours to ensure there are no irritations.

3. **Dampen a Cotton Pad:**

   - Take a cotton pad and dampen it with a small amount of the mixed oils. You want the pad to be moist but not dripping.

4. **Wipe Away Makeup:**

   ○ Gently wipe the damp cotton pad over your face, focusing on areas with makeup. The oils will work to dissolve the makeup, including waterproof products.

5. **Circular Motions:**

   ○ Use circular motions to help lift and remove the makeup effectively. Be gentle, especially around the delicate eye area.

6. **Rinse or Leave On (Optional):**

   ○ After makeup removal, you can either rinse your face with water or leave a thin layer of the oil mixture on your skin for added hydration. If you choose to leave it on, it acts as a moisturizing treatment.

7. **Follow with Cleanser (Optional):**

   ○ If desired, follow up with your regular facial cleanser to ensure all traces of makeup and oil are removed. This step is particularly important for those with oily or acne-prone skin.

8. **Store in a Cool Place:**

   ○ Keep the makeup remover in a cool, dark place. Ensure the container is tightly sealed to prevent oxidation.

Note: Adjust the oil ratios based on your skin type. Those with drier skin may prefer a slightly higher ratio of jojoba oil for added hydration, while those with oilier skin may lean towards a higher proportion of castor oil for its cleansing properties.

CHAPTER SEVENTEEN

Glossary

1. **Almond Oil (Sweet):**

   - Extracted from the kernels of sweet almonds (Prunus dulcis), this mild, hypoallergenic oil is known for its moisturizing and emollient properties.

2. **Argan Oil:**

   - Derived from the kernels of the argan tree (Argania spinosa), argan oil is rich in antioxidants and is known for its moisturizing effects.

3. **Avocado Oil:**

   - Obtained from the pulp of avocados, avocado oil is rich in fatty acids and is known for its moisturizing and nourishing properties.

4. **Baking Soda:**

- Sodium bicarbonate, a white crystalline powder commonly used for various household and personal care purposes.

5. **Beeswax:**

- A natural wax produced by honeybees, often used in skincare products for its emollient and protective properties.

6. **Black Pepper Oil:**

- Extracted from the dried fruits of Piper nigrum, black pepper oil is known for its spicy aroma and potential benefits for circulation.

7. **Castor Oil:**

- A vegetable oil obtained from the seeds of the castor bean (Ricinus communis), known for its moisturizing and anti-inflammatory properties.

8. **Coconut Oil:**

- Obtained from the meat of coconuts, coconut oil is a versatile oil with moisturizing properties commonly used in skincare and cooking.

9. **Egg Yolk:**

- The yellow part of an egg, often used in DIY skincare recipes for its nourishing and moisturizing properties.

10. **Eucalyptus Oil:**

   ○ Derived from the leaves of the eucalyptus tree, especially Eucalyptus globulus. It is known for its respiratory benefits and soothing properties.

11. **Ginger Oil:**

   ○ Obtained from the root of the ginger plant (Zingiber officinale), ginger oil has warming properties and is often used for its soothing effects.

12. **Glycerin:**

   ○ A humectant that attracts and retains moisture, glycerin is commonly used in skincare products for its hydrating properties.

13. **Hazel (Witch Hazel):**

   ○ Derived from the leaves and bark of the witch hazel plant (Hamamelis virginiana), witch hazel is a natural astringent with toning properties.

14. **Illipe Butter:**

   ○ Derived from the nuts of the Shorea stenoptera tree, illipe butter is a moisturizing and nourishing ingredient in skincare products.

15. **Jojoba Oil:**

   ○ Extracted from the seeds of the jojoba plant (Simmondsia chinensis), this oil closely resembles the skin's natural sebum. It is lightweight and non-comedogenic.

16. **Lavender Oil:**

- An essential oil extracted from lavender flowers (Lavandula angustifolia), known for its calming and soothing effects.

17. **Lemon:**

- A citrus fruit, and its essential oil is often used in skincare for its brightening and revitalizing properties.

18. **Marshmallow Extract:**

- Extracted from the root of the marshmallow plant (Althaea officinalis), marshmallow extract is known for its soothing and anti-inflammatory properties.

19. **Meadosweet:**

- A flowering plant whose extract is sometimes used in skincare for its potential anti-inflammatory and astringent properties.

20. **Mhyrr Essential Oil:**

- Extracted from the resin of the Commiphora myrrha tree, myrrh essential oil is known for its potential anti-inflammatory and soothing effects.

21. **Nettle Essential Oil:**

- Extracted from the leaves of the nettle plant, nettle essential oil is known for its potential benefits for the scalp and hair.

22. **Oat Milk:**

- A plant-based milk alternative made from oats, oat milk is sometimes used in skincare for its soothing properties.

23. **Olive Oil:**

- Extracted from olives, olive oil is a common cooking oil and is also used in skincare for its moisturizing properties.

24. **Orange Essential Oil:**

- Extracted from orange peels, orange essential oil is often used in skincare for its brightening and revitalizing properties.

25. **Papaya:**

- A tropical fruit whose fresh juice is sometimes used in skincare for its potential exfoliating and brightening properties.

26. **Peppermint Oil:**

- Extracted from the leaves of the peppermint plant (Mentha × piperita), peppermint oil provides a cooling and refreshing sensation.

27. **Pine Essential Oil:**

- Extracted from the needles of pine trees, pine essential oil is known for its potential benefits for oily skin.

28. **Pumpkin Seed Oil:**

- Obtained from pumpkin seeds, pumpkin seed oil is rich in vitamins and is used in skincare for its moisturizing and nourishing properties.

29. **Red Juniper Oil:**

- Extracted from the berries of the juniper tree, red juniper oil is sometimes used in skincare for its potential benefits for dry hair.

30. **Rosehip Oil:**

- Extracted from the seeds of rosehips, rosehip oil is known for its potential anti-aging and skin-renewing properties.

31. **Rosemary Oil:**

- Extracted from the leaves of the rosemary plant, rosemary oil is known for its potential benefits for the scalp and hair.

32. **Sage:**

- An herb whose essential oil is sometimes used in skincare for its potential benefits for oily skin.

33. **Sandalwood Oil:**

○ Extracted from the heartwood of sandalwood trees, sandalwood oil is known for its soothing and calming properties.

34. Sea Moss:

○ A type of seaweed or algae, sea moss is sometimes used in skincare for its potential hydrating properties.

35. Sesame Oil:

○ Extracted from sesame seeds, sesame oil is used in skincare for its moisturizing and antioxidant properties.

36. Shea Butter:

○ A fat extracted from the nuts of the shea tree (Vitellaria paradoxa). It is rich in fatty acids and has moisturizing and nourishing properties.

37. Sunflower Seed Oil:

○ Extracted from sunflower seeds, sunflower seed oil is used in skincare for its emollient and moisturizing properties.

38. Tea Tree Oil:

○ An essential oil derived from the leaves of the tea tree (Melaleuca alternifolia). It is known for its antimicrobial and anti-inflammatory properties.

39. Thyme Essential Oil:

- Extracted from the leaves of the thyme plant, thyme essential oil is known for its potential benefits for oily skin and hair.

40. **Vitamin E:**

- A fat-soluble vitamin often used in skincare for its antioxidant properties and ability to nourish the skin.

41. **Wheat Germ Oil:**

- Extracted from the germ of wheat kernels, wheat germ oil is rich in nutrients and is used in skincare for its potential benefits for dry skin and hair.

42. **Ylang Ylang Essential Oil:**

- Extracted from the flowers of the ylang-ylang tree, ylang-ylang essential oil is known for its sweet aroma and potential benefits for oily skin and hair.